T0245356

THE TOOTH AND NOTHING BUT THE TRUTH

A GERIATRIC DENTAL HYGIENIST AND GERIATRIC DENTIST'S GUIDE TO ORAL CARE FOR THE AGING POPULATION

SONYA DUNBAR, RDH, MHA
AND ALISA KAUFFMAN, DMD

AuthorHouse™
1663 Liberty Drive
Bloomington, IN 47403
www.authorhouse.com
Phone: 833-262-8899

Because of the dynamic nature of the Internet, any web addresses or links contained in this book may have changed
since publication and may no longer be valid. The views expressed in this work are solely those of the author and do
not necessarily reflect the views of the publisher, and the publisher hereby disclaims any responsibility for them.

Any people depicted in stock imagery provided by Getty Images are models,
and such images are being used for illustrative purposes only.
Certain stock imagery © Getty Images.

This book is printed on acid-free paper.

ISBN: 978-1-6655-2472-8 (sc)
978-1-6655-2473-5 (e)

Library of Congress Control Number: 2021908937

Print information available on the last page.

Published by AuthorHouse 05/17/2021

author HOUSE®

THE TOOTH AND NOTHING BUT THE TRUTH

A GERIATRIC DENTAL HYGIENIST AND GERIATRIC DENTIST'S GUIDE TO ORAL CARE FOR THE AGING POPULATION

Acknowledgments

Thank you, Dr. Berland and Willo, for creating products we love to recommend to our patients for their effectiveness and ease of use. And thank you to all our wonderful patients who make us love the career paths we both chose!

Sonya Dunbar RDH, MHA

I have been writing this book for over two years. In 2020 during the pandemic, I met Dr. Kauffman. Intrigued by her experience, I asked her to add some of her wisdom and insight to my journey. For over fifteen years, I have walked the halls of many long-term care facilities. I have been blessed to provide dental services to thousands of older adults. I have also helped improve the quality of life of elders at the end of their lives. As I offered dental care to these seniors, they were infusing me with wisdom for life.

I have learned that many seniors feel they become invisible as they age. I am fighting to improve oral health care for residents in long-term care facilities. That is my personal WHY for authoring this book. I am determined to "Be the voice for those whose voice has become a whisper."

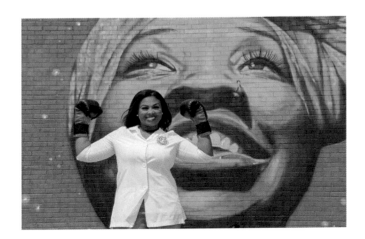

Dr. Alisa Kauffman

I wrote this book to honor my amazing mother, whom I spoke to five times a day about everything and nothing. She was always proud of my hard work and achievements. Sadly, my mother of sixty-one years, Theda Kauffman, passed away from complications of COVID-19 on August 26, 2020. I would also like to thank my father, husband, and daughter for always being there for me. And thank you to Sonya, my proud partner in new ventures. And as my mother loved to say, "Eat cake." Those two simple words put a quiet smile on my face. I will always love, honor, and cherish all the beautiful memories.

A few weeks after this painful event occurred, God sent me a gift in the form of a beautiful human being. Sonya Dunbar, the Geriatric Toothfairy, has become my newest dear friend/savior/confidant who has been there for me during this dark and painful time. She is teaching me how to mourn and how to continue living my life at the same time. Sonya gave me the greatest advice to help me get through this sad time in my life. I must keep myself busy in my work, as only time will heal this horrific wound.

When she asked me to co-author this book, I felt honored beyond words. We are both experts in this field, and we were meant to meet for this purpose. This book is intended to assist professionals in the geriatric field in maintaining patient oral health. Sonya is a pioneer in mobile services and a nationally recognized advocate for the geriatric population's oral care. And I have been practicing geriatric house call dentistry for over thirty-five years. Our ultimate goal is to improve aging adults' lives, specifically those in long-term care or those in need of house call care. As you age, we pray that you can continue to smile, be infection-free, and eat all the foods that make you happy. Eating cake was my mother's favorite food, and she enjoyed every bite!

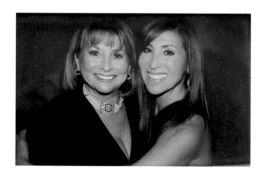

1-Elder Terminology and Demographics and Dental Terminology

Sonya Dunbar, the Geriatric Toothfairy

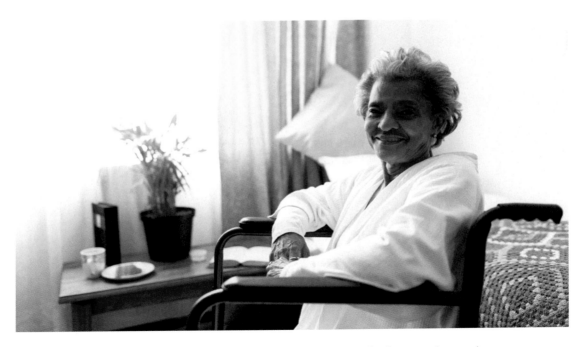

Before you enter into this world full of learning, knowledge, and wonder, you must be acquainted with specific older adult terminology and demographics.

wasn't always the Geriatric Toothfairy. This superpower and super passion took some time to brew and develop. I had a rough upbringing, but subtle rays of light lit up my life every summer that I spent with my grandmother, whom I affectionately called Madea. She was not just my grandmother; she was my mentor, my aspiration, my everything. I mean, how many teens do you know who enjoy the company of someone forty years older than they are? Well, I did, and so did many of my friends.

After I got my red 1982 Ford Escort at the age of sixteen, I would go pick her up, and we would hang out, laugh, and talk. Madea instilled so much wisdom into me. Though her delivery was not as formal as this book is, I would like to impart some of those golden nuggets of infinite wisdom to you.

Before you enter into this world full of learning, knowledge, and wonder, preparation is needed. You must become acquainted with specific older-adult terminology and demographics as well as dental terminology. Some vocabulary terms may be unknown or different from what you are accustomed to. In case you didn't know, "elder" is an honorable term, and "elderly" isn't as honorable. I respect, admire, and uphold my elders because they are the world's wise men and women. I believe that they should be regarded as such.

Elder Terminology

- **Elders** are older adults born between 1946 and 1964.

- **Geriatrics** is an area of medicine concerned with the illnesses of old age and their treatments. This field's primary goals are to promote elders' health and prevent and treat diseases that they may encounter after a certain age.

- **Gerontology** is the scientific study of the factors that affect the normal aging process and the effect of aging. It accesses physical, mental, and social changes in people as they grow older. This knowledge can then be applied to policies and programs throughout the world.

- **Chronologic age** is age measured by calendar time since birth and, therefore, the actual amount of time that a person has been alive.

- **Functional age** is age based on capabilities to maintain activities. A person may show the benefits and behaviors of a particular age group that may not be anywhere near their chronological age.

- **Activities of daily living (ADLs)** collectively describe fundamental skills required to independently care for oneself, such as eating, bathing, and mobility.

- **Candida** is yeast often found in association with oral disease, such as thrush.

- **Calculus, or tartar**, is a hard deposit attached to the teeth, usually consisting of mineralized bacterial plaque.

- **Dental hygienists** are licensed professional dental auxiliaries who are both oral health educators and clinicians and use preventive, educational, and therapeutic methods to control oral disease.

- **Dental plaque** is a sticky, colorless film that constantly forms on the teeth. The bacteria in dental plaque cause periodontal disease. If plaque is not removed carefully each day by brushing and flossing, it becomes calculus.

- **Dentures** are artificial substitutes for missing natural teeth. A complete denture replaces all of the teeth in an arch.[1]

Now that you know these terms, I feel comfortable inviting you into a fairyland where the world of dental hygiene meets the forgotten generation.

Older-Adult Demographics

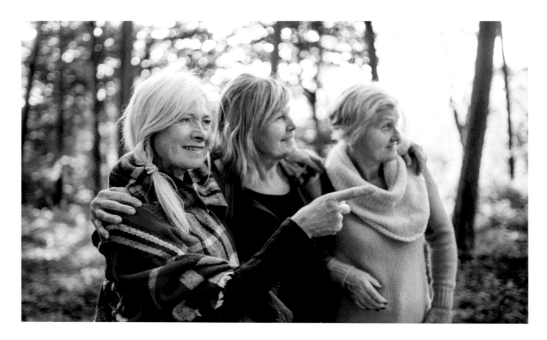

The youngest baby boomer is about sixty-five years old, and the eldest is about eighty-four.

The 2020 census estimated the baby boomer generation at 73 million.[2] The youngest baby boomer is about sixty-five years old; the eldest is about eighty-four. While this generation is known to have higher education than their ancestors, they experience more significant economic disparities. According to the US Census Bureau, aging adults are working much longer than their ancestors, which has increased their life expectancy.

The oral health of older adults is important because the number of US adults aged sixty-five years or older is expected to reach 98 million by 2060.[3] Older adults, especially those who are economically disadvantaged, lack insurance, or are members of racial and ethnic minorities tend to have poor oral health. Being disabled, homebound, or institutionalized (e.g., living in a nursing home) also increases the risk of poor oral health. Besides, many older adults do not have dental insurance because they lost their benefits upon retirement, and the federal Medicare program does not cover routine dental care.[4]

2—Why Do People End Up in Long-Term Care Facilities?

Sonya Dunbar, the Geriatric Toothfairy

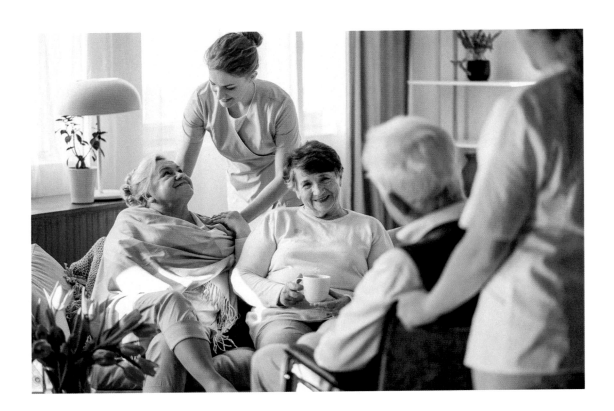

have always loved smiling. When I was much younger, I created the stare-and-smile game, where I would stare at people until they cracked a smile. I fell in love with capturing smiles at a young age, and I continue to love the warm feeling it gives me. Madea would always say that a smile is something that you can give away and still keep for yourself. These nuggets of wisdom made me who I am today.

Like the tooth fairy, I am dedicated to specific age groups. I do not leave money under pillows, but I do fly around the world, serving the elder community and voicing the issues and concerns often not addressed. Geriatric care focuses on baby boomers, who were born between 1946 and 1964. This generation makes up a large portion of the population of the world because the number of babies born "boomed" after the Second World War and continued to rise until the 1960s.[5] They now represent nearly 20 percent of the American public.[6] That is why understanding older adults' health is becoming increasingly essential. Geriatrics and gerontology have become integral pieces for preparing for the future.

Moving In with Adult Children and Other Family Members

In some cases, aging first begins with elders leaving their own homes to live with their children or other family members. Guilt and underestimation are contributing factors to making such a decision. Families want to ensure that their parents are happy and comfortable. It is assumed that living with them will be the best option to achieve that goal.

However, the demands of senior care can become overwhelming over time and are something that many caregivers fail to foresee. The demands may include managing medications, keeping track of doctors' appointments, coping with changes in behavior, and helping elders with daily living activities. Feeling underqualified and overwhelmed often leads to the decision to put loved ones in long-term care facilities with professional staff providing around-the-clock care. This is more practical for all parties involved.

Moving into Long-Term Care Is the New Normal

Before I was forced to put my grandmother in a nursing home, I always assumed that putting your loved one in a long-term care facility was a decision to neglect your family member. That couldn't have been further from the truth. The reality is people tend to end up in long-term care facilities when completing activities of daily living (ADLs) becomes problematic, primarily bathing, toileting, transferring oneself, eating, dressing, and ambulating.

In table 1, the different ADLs that become a challenge to seniors as they age are listed and defined. A report published by the US Department of Health and Human Services found that people aged sixty-five and older have a strong chance—70 percent—of needing long-term care.[4] Despite this high rate, many caregivers and loved ones do not plan for such things. Moving into long-term care is the new normal for elders.

Table 1

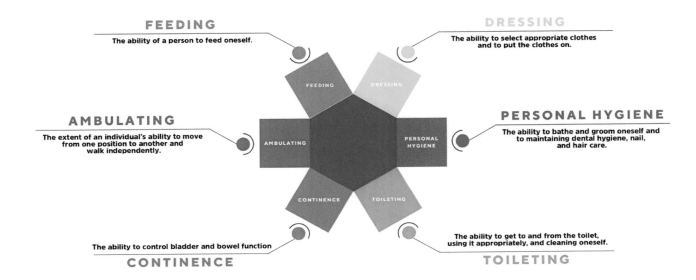

Challenging ADL's

FEEDING
The ability of a person to feed oneself.

DRESSING
The ability to select appropriate clothes and to put the clothes on.

AMBULATING
The extent of an individual's ability to move from one position to another and walk independently.

PERSONAL HYGIENE
The ability to bathe and groom oneself and to maintaining dental hygiene, nail, and hair care.

CONTINENCE
The ability to control bladder and bowel function

TOILETING
The ability to get to and from the toilet, using it appropriately, and cleaning oneself.

Caregivers in Long-Term Care Facilities

Sonya Dunbar, The Geriatric Toothfairy

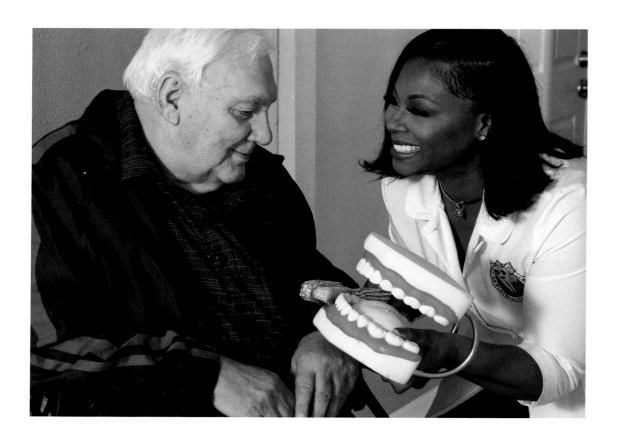

Growing up around Madea gave me a deeper appreciation for aging adults, specifically in long-term care facilities. I promised my grandmother when I was younger that I would never put her in a nursing home. That was a promise I could not keep. As her health began to decline, I decided it would be best to move her into my house with me. She lived with me for a while, but it got to a point where I felt that she would get better care for her illnesses elsewhere. She developed type 2 diabetes, which led to the amputation of one of her legs, and she was not able to complete ADLs independently.

After making the big decision to place my grandmother into a long-term facility, I vowed that I would not go more than a couple of days without visiting her. I stuck to this oath. On my best week, I would see Madea every single day. I could not help but notice that her oral care was being neglected. At times I would take out her dentures and see all of the food she had eaten the day before. That was a no-no! As you can imagine, I was livid.

I had a few words with her assigned certified nursing assistant (CNA) and quickly realized that she was not neglecting any of her patients on purpose. She simply did not know that my grandmother had dentures, and she did not know how to take them out. I had grown a deep appreciation for CNAs and caregivers because I worked alongside them and was introduced to what goes on behind the scenes. I knew then that I was also responsible for ensuring that Madea had proper oral care. I felt responsible for educating her CNAs on proper oral care.

Responsibilities of Carers and Nurses

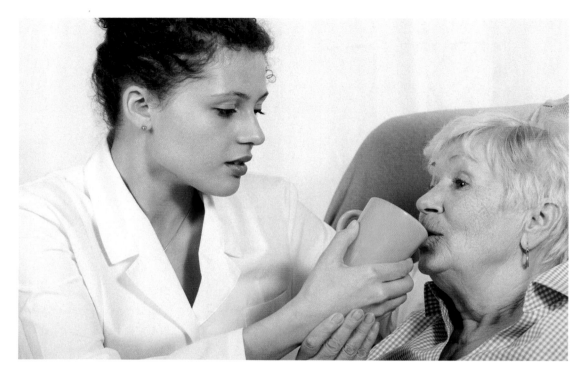

Caring for those who once cared for us in the highest honor.
—Tia Walker

CNAs are the primary caregivers in such facilities. Their duties relate directly to hands-on care and patient support. A standard shift may involve handling phone calls, helping patients with daily and physical activities, changing beds, and keeping an eye on their food consumption. Daily and physical activities include serving and assisting senior patients with ADLs, maintaining patient hygiene and nutrition, and managing residents' medication. They are mostly responsible for the residents' health and safety under the supervision of a nurse.

They are also tasked with ensuring that patients are getting proper nutrition from food and vitamins. With a task list this long and a heavy patient load coupled with being grossly underpaid, it is no wonder why so many CNAs are stressed and pushed to the limit.

Challenges of CNAs

- Nursing assistants are three and a half times more likely to be injured on the job than the typical US worker.

- Wages for CNAs have not kept up with inflation over the past ten years: inflation-adjusted wages remained relatively stagnant, decreasing from $12.22 in 2005 to $11.87 in 2015.

- More than half of CNAs work part time or for part of the year. As a result of low wages and part-time work hours, CNAs in this industry earn a median annual income of $19,000 a year.

- Low annual earnings result in a relatively high rate of poverty among CNAs: 17 percent live below the federal poverty line, compared to 9 percent of all US workers.

- Because poverty rates are high among CNAs, nearly 40 percent rely on some form of public assistance.

- CNAs outnumber any other occupation employed in nursing homes by a factor of at least three to one. The number of CNAs, 612,000, has remained relatively constant over the past ten years.

- CNAs spend more time than any other nursing staff assisting residents, providing a median of 2.4 hours of hands-on care per resident every day. Their frequent interactions with residents enable them to observe changes in residents' condition and report these changes to licensed nursing staff.

- From 2014 to 2024, CNAs will contribute more to nursing home employment growth than any other occupation. Of total employment growth across the industry, new CNA jobs will comprise 39 percent.[7]

Caregiver Training

Senior caregivers have a heavy influence on the happiness and well-being of the patient. The better their experience is with the caregivers, the happier they will be. Most care facilities standards call for at least one licensed nurse for every forty residents in their custody. Most

CNAs are required to take an auditory learning course between four and twelve weeks and must be well aware of the basics when caring for the facility's residents. As you could imagine, this is quite a bit to learn in such a short amount of time. Exhibit 2 illustrates the many topics that most CNA courses cover. The specific topics vary from state to state.

Typically most CNA programs are divided into two parts: contact hours and clinic practice. State-approved programs offer a minimum of seventy-five hours of classroom instruction and clinical training.[8] That is less than four days of training that caregivers mostly between the ages of twenty-five and thirty-five years old learn how to properly care for patients who are double and sometimes triple their age. Do you notice what the problem is yet?[68] Specifically:

- The CNA-to-patient ratio is one to twenty.

- Licensed nurses must provide a minimum of one hour a day in direct service to residents.

- A facility must have at least one licensed nurse for every forty residents.

It is no secret that most caregivers feel overwhelmed and undertrained for their job descriptions, which often entail duties not written on paper. The need for caregiver support in the senior community is tremendous. There must be more support and training for this workforce. Low competition for CNAs makes it difficult to keep the positions filled. There is a rapid turnover rate. With older Americans living longer, it is imperative to develop strategies to stabilize and strengthen this workforce.

Outside Caregivers

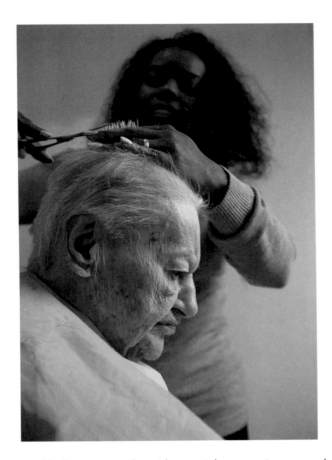

Seniors are more likely to comply with outside caregivers, such as a spouse
or adult child, because they are more familiar with them.

An outside caregiver provides care and emotional support for a resident without working for the care facility. The person could be a spouse or adult child who visits regularly. Outside caregivers are essential because:

- Patients are typically more compliant with outside caregivers than in-house caregivers because of familiarity.

- Outside caregivers are often the voices for mute and faint seniors. They have the intuition to observe and address changes in residents' behavior.

- Outside caregivers provide emotional support for long-term care residents.

- Outside caregivers, like mobile and teledentistry personnel, can lower the workload of the understaffed nurses, which prevents staff burnout.

- Loved ones who are active in facilities maintain a sense of continuity and identity for residents.

However, since March 2020, restrictions have been in place in these long-term care facilities to reduce visitor numbers. Recognizing the critical role of outside caregivers has been a big focus throughout the coronavirus pandemic since long-term separation and isolation can negatively affect residents' health.[9]

Summary

CNAs are the primary caregivers of seniors in long-term care facilities. Most CNAs are required to take an auditory learning course that takes four to twelve weeks. They must be well aware of the basics when caring for the facility's residents. Most care facilities standards call for at least one licensed nurse for every forty residents in their custody. As a result, many of the caregivers are overwhelmed. An outside caregiver can help take care of seniors, offer emotional support, and speak for them.

3—Importance of Social Skills for Seniors

Sonya Dunbar, the Geriatric Toothfairy

t took months for my grandmother and me to adjust to the new life we were both living. Though she was a longtime resident of a senior living facility, I became a long-term outside caregiver of that facility. I did not realize it then, but she was my first patient. I tried my best to come prepared. Weeks passed by, and I became my grandmother's primary oral health caregiver. I will never forget when I heard Madea's roommate speak to me for the first time. Every time I came into their room, she stared but never talked to me, even when I spoke to her. I knew she was a sweet lady, as Madea told me so.

She motioned me to come over to her, and I did.

I bent down, and she said in the sweetest voice, "Baby, can you clean my teeth? Mine don't come out like your grandmother's do."

I was happy to oblige, but I had one problem. I couldn't find her toothbrush anywhere in her room. From that day on, I purposed in my heart to bring a toothbrush with me every time that I set foot on that nursing home property.

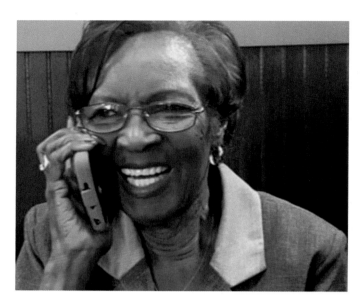

Elders socialize at long-term care facilities. A happy life is impossible without good health and vice versa.

Being social is vital to elders because social activities keep seniors sharp and mentally engaged; help prevent dementia or Alzheimer's disease; improves senior physical health, which boosts the immune system; and encourages better sleep patterns, which promotes longer life.

Social engagement is considered to be an active activity for aging adults. They may go out for a walk with a family member or anything. Without this, aging adults may not have much reason to leave the house or be active in any way. A happy life is impossible without good health and vice versa.

Neglected oral health affects a senior's overall health and quality of life. Oral neglect includes chipped teeth, ill-fitting dentures, and decaying teeth that are brittle and tend to fall out easily. The consequences of decayed teeth or ill-fitting dentures can drastically alter how a person acts and lives. Not only do they feel extremely uncomfortable, but they won't feel like doing much or interacting with others. Seniors will isolate themselves, which results in a nonexistent social life. The lack of social interaction can lead to more deep-rooted problems like depression and loneliness.

Depression affects around 6 million Americans at ages sixty-five and over. Only 10 percent of these people receive treatment despite it also being associated with an increased risk of death after a heart attack or illness.[10] It is vital to be mindful of the direct connection between senior's oral and mental health. Researchers have found that adults suffering from severe mental illnesses are more likely to have poor oral health. According to data, 60 percent of people with mental health issues also have poor oral health.[11] Having decayed teeth or bad breath can also drastically affect self-esteem, and the pain could lead to lack of sleep and not being able to eat correctly. All these factors are why keeping our elders healthy—physically, orally, and mentally—is important. Alzheimer's disease can lead to difficulty swallowing, chewing, moving, weight loss, and memory loss.

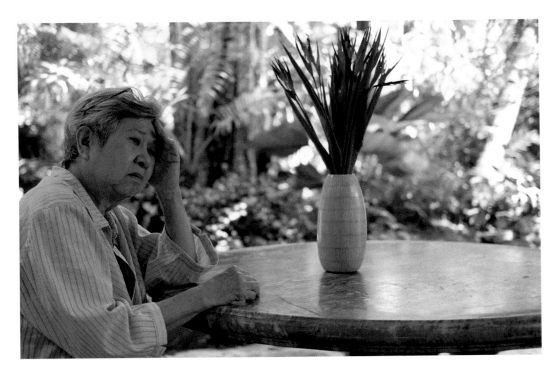

Seniors with decayed teeth and ill-fitting dentures feel extremely uncomfortable and won't feel like doing much or interacting with others.

Recognizing Victims of Poor Oral Health

Socialization is the activity of mixing socially with others. It's intended to foster relationships, establish good communication skills, and promote a sense of community.[12] The value of socialization never disappears, and it's particularly relevant for seniors because socializing keeps people young at heart, emotionally alive, and sharp mentally.

Have you taken the time to consider the continued importance of socialization for your aging parent or loved one? Parents recognize the importance of encouraging socialization in their children's development to enhance lifestyle and expose them to new experiences. It is the same concept as our seniors. They need new experiences and to continually learn new things. Socialization continues to build character as seniors are challenged and intrigued by conversation and collaborative activities.

Learning to work together in board games can translate to seniors helping their roommates and others around them in everyday life situations. Socialization ensures that aging adults maintain a healthy physical and emotional balance.

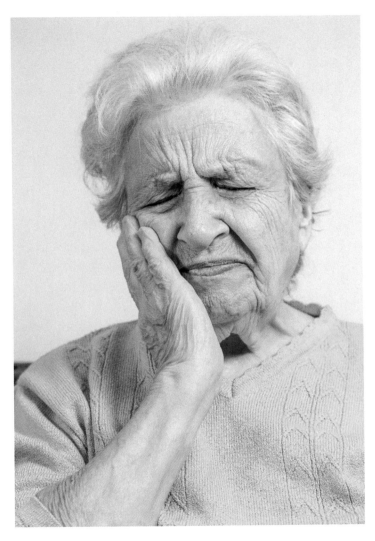

If a senior fails to communicate discomfort, it is the caregiver's responsibility to read the signs.

Social skills in senior lifestyle are essential, but what happens when you run across a senior who is not social? Grumpiness could be a possibility, but poor oral health is a greater possibility. It is not foreign to encounter patients plagued with dementia or find it challenging to communicate with caregivers. If the patient fails to communicate discomfort, it is the caregiver's responsibility to read poor oral health signs. Some of those symptoms include a refusal to eat; a pulling at the face or mouth; leaving dentures out; increased restlessness, moaning, or shouting; disturbed sleep; a refusal to participate in activities; or increased aggression.

The name of the game is awareness. In-house and outside care providers must recognize that the symptoms listed previously could be a product of tooth decay. Surveyors have determined that 96 percent of aging adults sixty-five or older have had a cavity and one in five have untreated tooth decay. Untreated temporary ailments turn into life-threatening diseases.

Summary

It is important for seniors to socialize as it increases their quality of life. However, they might not be comfortable enough to engage in social activities when they are suffering from poor oral health. Lack of socialization may lead to isolation and depression, which may result in death. If caregivers look out for symptoms of poor oral health and help them seek treatment, this will aid them in avoiding life-threatening diseases and being able to socialize again.

4—Preventing Oral Neglect in Aging Communities

Sonya Dunbar, the Geriatric Toothfairy

Once I had a hundred-year-old patient whom I deemed to be mute. She would greet me with a nice, big smile. I talked and cracked jokes, trying to keep her smiling every visit. I adored her. I gave her detailed instructions on how to improve her oral health each visit for at least a year. One day after finishing up a routine cleaning, I was wheeling this patient back to her room, and she motioned me to slow down. It turns out she recognized the pastor walking down the hallway.

As I slowed down, my patient spoke out in a firm voice. I stood there in shock as she conversed with the pastor and giggled at all of his jokes. I learned something valuable that day. My patient saw me as an ordinary caregiver. She was guarded and did not feel comfortable enough to talk to me. Weeks later, that changed. Neglect has a toll on patients, leaving dental professionals responsible for combatting oral neglect.

Providing Oral Care in Facilities

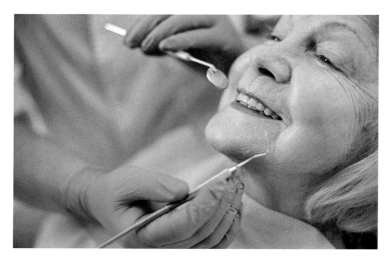

Dental professionals should examine the residents upon their admission to long-term care facilities and offer regular reviews to diagnose and treat oral diseases.

Facilities need to provide adequate oral care to seniors to maintain their health and well-being. This includes having a dental professional examine the residents upon their admission to diagnose oral diseases, such as oral and dental cavities and periodontal disease, and administer treatment.[32]

A dental professional should also be involved in creating an oral care plan for the elders when they join the facility. The plan should be based on the senior's level of oral health and their ability to independently perform daily oral hygiene procedures, such as brushing their teeth.[13] Adequate daily oral care and regular review by dental professionals will help prevent the progression of dental disease, improve the physical functioning of the teeth, and reduce pneumonia-related complications.[14]

Educating Residents and Staff

As a person ages, it becomes harder for them to take care of themselves. It is, therefore, important to educate and promote awareness about the importance of oral care to seniors and their caregivers.[15] This could help prevent oral diseases and complications. For example, some seniors do not remove their dentures because they do not remember or fear that they could be stolen or the staff does not know how to do it. Not removing dentures could cause complications, such as oral thrush, odors, and irritation. Offering education on the importance of removing dentures and other oral hygiene procedures will reduce such complications.

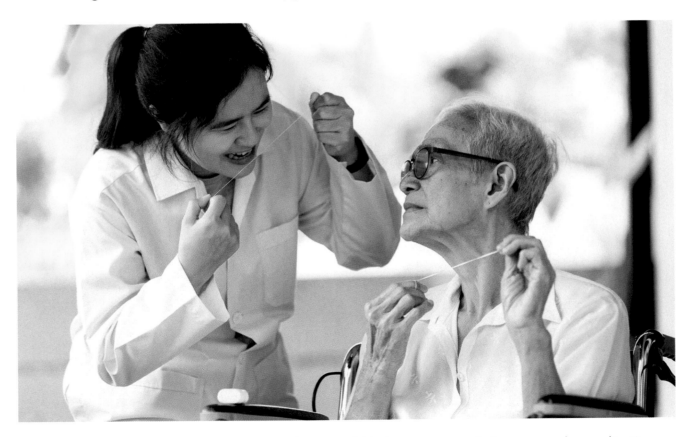

Educating seniors on oral hygiene procedures could help prevent oral diseases and complications.

Facilities should also transfer knowledge on oral health to the staff, mostly CNAs, who take care of seniors in long-term care facilities. Studies show that a majority of staff in these facilities have received inadequate training in oral care procedures, such as brushing, flossing, and cleaning dentures.[16] Training them on these oral care procedures will help build their competence and confidence to offer better oral care to the seniors.[17] This will help prevent premature death of seniors, most of whom die from systemic diseases directly linked to oral care, such as aspiration pneumonia, heart disease, cancer, urinary tract infection, and Alzheimer's disease.

Bringing Community Awareness

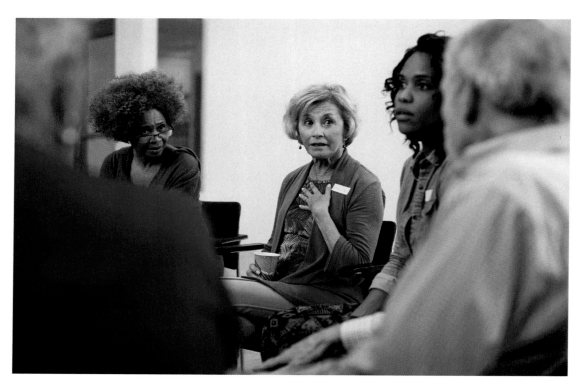

Members of the community should bring awareness about the impact of aging on oral health.

A significant barrier to oral health care of seniors is the underestimation of the oral care that they need.[17] Community members, including dental professionals, academics, and policymakers, need to raise awareness about the need for equity in the provision of oral health,[18] for instance, the impact of aging on oral health and the need for proper daily and professional care for seniors and funding resources of oral health-care programs of seniors.[19]

Community members can spread this knowledge using different methods, including direct communication during office visits, written messages, seminars, and mass media. Building community awareness in addition to providing adequate oral health care in aging facilities will help improve oral health care of seniors.[20]

Summary

Long-term care facilities need to provide adequate oral care to ensure the well-being of seniors. This includes having a dentist examine the seniors upon admission, helping develop an oral care plan for them, and offering regular oral exams. To improve the health of seniors, it is also important to educate residents and staff to help build their capacity and confidence to offer better oral care to elders. Additionally, members of the community need to raise awareness about the impact of aging on oral health as well as the need for daily and professional oral care for seniors and resources. Raising awareness and providing oral health care will help improve the oral care of seniors.

5—Oral Care Preventatives

Sonya Dunbar, the Geriatric Toothfairy

Madea adjusted to the nursing home quite well. She was a social butterfly. She became the talk of the home. I will never forget coming to visit her one day and being met at her door with lines of elders, surprisingly waiting for me in her room. As I greeted everyone and worked my way through the crowd and into her room, I was shocked to hear from her roommate that she wasn't there and that she had stepped outside for a "smoke break."

My grandmother wore an oxygen mask. I just knew that this was a joke. But, sure enough, when I stepped out onto the courtyard there, she was with her oxygen mask cocked to the side, smoking a cigarette. I went over to her laughing the whole way over in true disbelief. I asked her how she got outside and where she got the cigarettes. She told me that she had promised her home mates that I would clean their teeth. Can you believe it? She was bartering me out for a cigarette. I thought I was worth at least a whole pack.

I gained almost a whole floor of unofficial patients overnight thanks to Madea's bartering deal. I got the pleasure of assisting a sweet lady who suffered from dementia. In addition to not knowing where her toothbrush was, she also forgot to brush her teeth. Though she was a sweet lady, she could easily be labeled as challenging because it took her some time to warm up to me each time I visited her. I realized that patients who have Alzheimer's or any of the like are more likely to experience oral neglect because they may forget to brush or how to use a toothbrush or they may not be able to express pain or oral concern to caregivers.

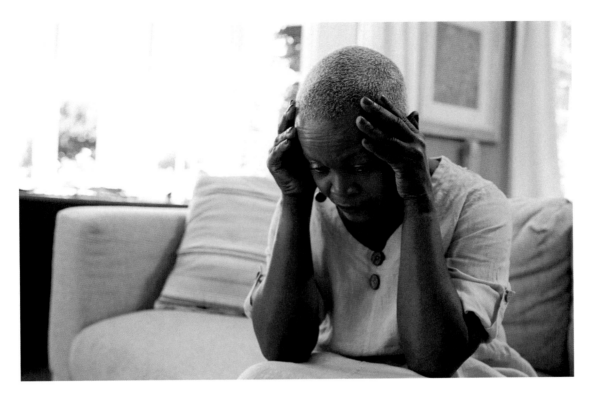

An elder suffering from memory loss, an oral care preventive.

Elders who suffer from dexterity and arthritis are at risk for poor oral care. It has been assumed that since arthritis is common, patients are accustomed to the side effects that come with the ailment. That couldn't be the furthest thing from the truth. The truth is that arthritis is a broad spectrum and there are levels to the pain and preventions. Though arthritis can be seen physically with the naked eye, an x-ray can only detect the severity of it. The x-ray machine picks up symptoms like enlarged and inflamed joints. Inflammation in the joints can prevent aging adults from performing ADLs. The simplest tasks become complicated. When dexterity is compromised, the patient cannot tend to their oral health daily. Inevitably they suffer.

Dementia and memory loss are also oral care preventives. Studies have shown that there is a direct link to dementia and gingivitis. A recent study has determined that the bacteria that causes gingivitis also may be connected to Alzheimer's disease. Scientists have previously found that this species of bacteria, Porphyromonas gingivalis, can move from the mouth to the brain. Once in the brain, the bacteria release enzymes called gingipains that can destroy nerve cells, which in turn can lead to memory loss and eventually Alzheimer's. When aging adults start losing their memory, they cannot remember small things like brushing their teeth, bathing, or eating that day. The lack of memory, among many other factors, leads to poor oral health.

Researchers surveyed the oral health of 987 people living in aged residential care and found those with dementia, and older men in general, have dirtier and more decayed teeth. Head of the Department of Oral Sciences at the University of Otago and lead author of the study describes poor oral health as one of the "geriatric giants" with the situation a "major clinical and public health problem which is going to get worse."

Aging adults have higher cognitive and physical impairments that can adversely affect their oral self-care and complicate oral care provision. About half of those examined in the study had severely impaired cognitive function, and more than a third required fillings or extractions. Those with severely damaged cognitive function had greater numbers of teeth with decay and higher oral debris scores, reflecting deficient daily oral hygiene. Greater rates of tooth decay can result in dental and facial infections, lower quality of life, malnutrition, and communication difficulties.[21]

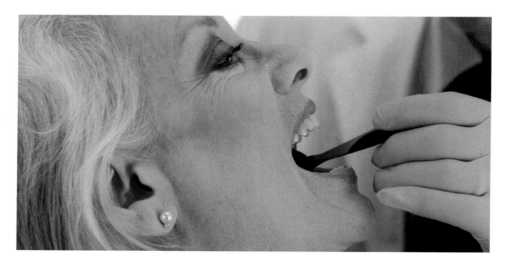

A dental professional implementing preventative care on a senior to eliminate the need for extensive procedures later when the patient may be less able to tolerate it.

When dental professionals encounter patients who already have Alzheimer's, their goal should be to implement preventative care such as plaque removal, scaling, flossing, and fluoride varnish application. These procedures are performed to eliminate the need for extensive procedures later on, when patients with dementia may be less able to tolerate them. During the middle and late stages of Alzheimer's, oral health may become more challenging. The person may forget what to do with toothpaste or how to rinse or be resistant to others' assistance. This forgetfulness leads to neglect, which leads to diseases.

It is estimated that 71 million Americans, approximately 20 percent of the population, will be sixty-five years or older by 2030. An increasing number of older persons have some or all of their teeth intact because of improvements in oral health care, such as community water fluoridation, advanced dental technology, and better oral hygiene. Nevertheless, the greatest generation is at risk of the mouth's chronic diseases. These diseases include Caries, periodontitis, gingivitis, and xerostomia.[22]

Preventative Measures to Adopt in Daily Senior Care

Fluoride gels, rinses, and varnishes may prevent or reduce root caries. Patients with xerostomia should be encouraged to drink water and avoid products that contain alcohol as well as foods and drinks that contain sugar. Over-the-counter saliva substitutes are encouraged. Topical antifungal therapies are effective for treating denture stomatitis and angular cheilitis caused by candidiasis.

Exhibit 2 further illustrates common oral conditions that contribute to barriers in senior oral care. Notice that most of these conditions can be avoided with professional dental intervention, being that these conditions are painful, and paired with limited ADL abilities, patients depend on dental professionals and caregivers to administer preventative care because many seniors have the ability to.

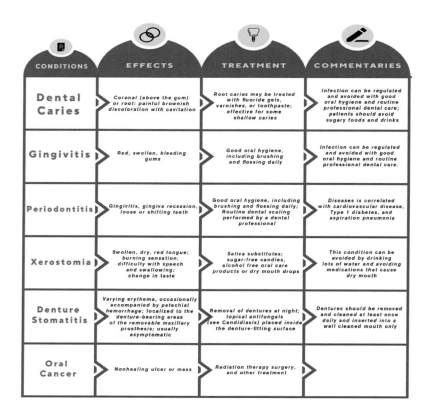

Conditional Oral Care Barriers

CONDITIONS	EFFECTS	TREATMENT	COMMENTARIES
Dental Caries	Coronal (above the gum) or root: painful brownish discoloration with cavitation	Root caries may be treated with fluoride gels, varnishes, or toothpaste; effective for some shallow caries	Infection can be regulated and avoided with good oral hygiene and routine professional dental care; patients should avoid sugary foods and drinks
Gingivitis	Red, swollen, bleeding gums	Good oral hygiene, including brushing and flossing daily	Infection can be regulated and avoided with good oral hygiene and routine professional dental care.
Periodontitis	Gingivitis, gingiva recession, loose or shifting teeth	Good oral hygiene, including brushing and flossing daily; Routine dental scaling performed by a dental professional	Diseases is correlated with cardiovascular disease, Type 1 diabetes, and aspiration pneumonia
Xerostomia	Swollen, dry, red tongue; burning sensation; difficulty with speech and swallowing; change in taste	Saliva substitutes; sugar-free candies, alcohol free oral care products or dry mouth drops	This condition can be avoided by drinking lots of water and avoiding medications that cause dry mouth
Denture Stomatitis	Varying erythema, occasionally accompanied by petechial hemorrhage; localized to the denture-bearing areas of the removable maxillary prosthesis; usually asymptomatic	Removal of dentures at night; topical antifungals (see Candidiasis) placed inside the denture-fitting surface	Dentures should be removed and cleaned at least once daily and inserted into a well cleaned mouth only
Oral Cancer	Nonhealing ulcer or mass	Radiation therapy surgery, and other treatment	

Summary

Elders who suffer from diseases such as Alzheimer's, dexterity issues, arthritis, and others that cause pain or memory loss are at risk of poor oral health because they are unable to personally tend to their oral care needs, are in constant pain, or cannot express their concerns to caregivers. When dental professionals encounter elders with such conditions, their goal should be implementing preventative care, such as plaque removal, scaling, flossing, and fluoride varnish application. These treatments will eliminate the need for extensive procedures later, when patients are less likely to tolerate them.

6—Medications

Sonya Dunbar, the Geriatric Toothfairy

Medication is the reason I decided that it would be best to put my grandmother in long-term care. The fear of giving her the wrong medication at the wrong time by mistake made the decision much easier. The average number of medications for each resident in long-term care is 9.7 per day! With three children, a husband, and a full-time job, I knew it was impossible to be error-free when it came to anything. Being the primary caregiver of anyone takes attention to detail and a clear head.

At the time, that was something I lacked. I later was informed by observing Madea that I made the right decision. Doctors were able to anticipate her needs and connect the dots between her ailments and oral health. I learned a lot about how medications affect the mouth during that time.

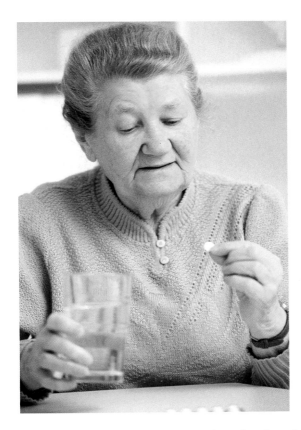

The aging process affects how medications are absorbed and used in the body.

Effect of Medication on Teeth

Medications can be tricky when paired with the aging body. There are side effects that occur as soon as the medication is taken until it leaves the body. The aging process affects how medications are absorbed, used in the body, and exit the body. Digestion plays a key role in determining how fast or slow these processes go. Slow digestion decreases the body's ability to break down and eliminate certain medications. For these reasons, lower doses are recommended for seniors. According to the American Geriatrics Society, several precautions need to be taken when seniors are taking medication.

When taking medications, it is essential to make sure that the correct medication is prescribed for the correct condition, the medication is age-appropriate, and the proper dose is prescribed for the length of time.

Many ailments like asthma, gum disease, arthritis, and chronic immune deficiencies cause daily medication dosages. Over time, the ingredients in the medications taken, combined with poor oral care, lead to other side effects. Most drugs that affect the immune system also trigger the overgrowth of the fungus Candida albicans in the mouth. Aging in and of itself does not automatically lead to all ailments and mouth malfunctions.

Aging does impair the sense of taste. Diseases, medications, and dentures can contribute to this sensory loss. Given the difficulty seniors face performing certain medical conditions, that makes proper oral care challenging to perform independently. Arthritis in the hands and fingers may make brushing or flossing teeth difficult to impossible to perform without medication.

Exhibit 3 illustrates different medications that affect the mouth.

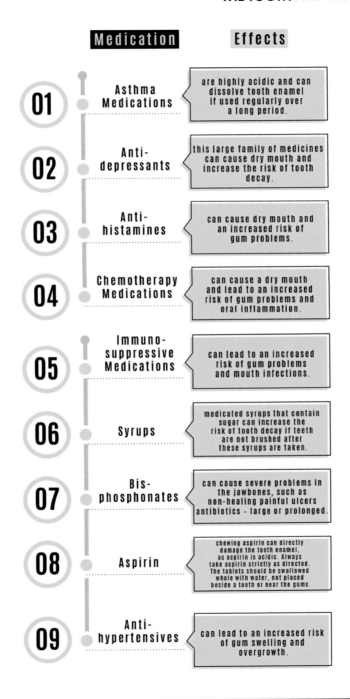

Medication	Effects
01 Asthma Medications	are highly acidic and can dissolve tooth enamel if used regularly over a long period.
02 Anti-depressants	this large family of medicines can cause dry mouth and increase the risk of tooth decay.
03 Anti-histamines	can cause dry mouth and an increased risk of gum problems.
04 Chemotherapy Medications	can cause a dry mouth and lead to an increased risk of gum problems and oral inflammation.
05 Immuno-suppressive Medications	can lead to an increased risk of gum problems and mouth infections.
06 Syrups	medicated syrups that contain sugar can increase the risk of tooth decay if teeth are not brushed after these syrups are taken.
07 Bis-phosphonates	can cause severe problems in the jawbones, such as non-healing painful ulcers antibiotics - large or prolonged.
08 Aspirin	chewing aspirin can directly damage the tooth enamel, as aspirin is acidic. Always take aspirin strictly as directed. The tablets should be swallowed whole with water, not placed beside a tooth or near the gums.
09 Anti-hypertensives	can lead to an increased risk of gum swelling and overgrowth.

Years ago, medications for seniors in long-term care facilities were limited. Pills were few, and basic syrups were given to them for minor colds, headaches, and common body aches. Many of the more complicated ailments that they suffered from were deemed to be terminal illnesses. Things have changed since then, and there are more medications and options for seniors. These medications have contributed to a longer and fuller life for many aging adults. Unfortunately this gift of medicine comes with some side effects. Studies have shown to be just as detrimental as the illness treated if the caregiver and dental professionals are unaware of the side effects and the proper methods to combat them.

Proper tongue care for all patients, but especially those administered medications daily, is pertinent to patient health and longevity. Most patients cannot take pills whole, so caregivers crush them up and feed them to patients, leaving pill residue on their tongues. Suppose seniors are not receiving daily oral care. The medication begins to have unintended side effects like altering their sense of taste and causing dry mouth and foul odors.

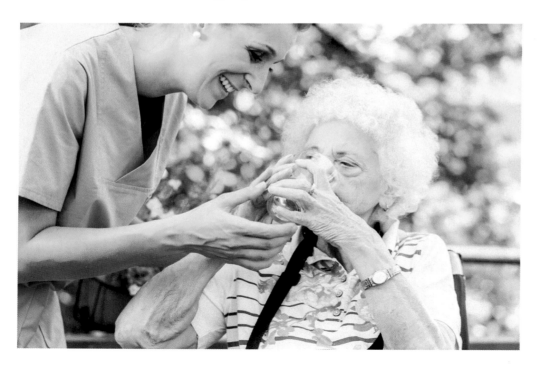

Dry mouth, a side effect of more than five hundred medications, is painful.

Dry Mouth

Saliva is the mouth's primary defense against tooth decay. Saliva maintains the health of the soft and hard tissues in the mouth. It washes away food and other debris, neutralizes acids produced by bacteria in the mouth, and provides disease-fighting substances throughout the mouth, offering first-line protection against microbial invasion or overgrowth that might lead to disease. In a recent and comprehensive national survey of US noninstitutionalized adults, it was reported that more than 90 percent of people sixty-five or older use at least one medication per week; more than 40 percent of this population use five or more different medications per week; and 12 percent use ten or more different medications per week. Many of these medications cause dry mouth.

Dry mouth—also called xerostomia—results from an inadequate flow of saliva. Dry mouth is not a normal part of aging. However, it is a side effect in more than five hundred medications, including those for allergies or asthma, high blood pressure, high cholesterol, pain, anxiety or depression, Parkinson's, and Alzheimer's diseases.

As you could imagine, dry mouth is painful. Dental professionals are encouraged to prescribe medication that does not cause dry mouth. Patients are encouraged to choose sugar-free candies and gums as well as alcohol-free dental products. Saliva substitutes are also a very popular solution to dry mouth. Many seniors frequent medications that they need to live.

Summary

Seniors take several medications for ailments, such as asthma, gum disease, arthritis, and chronic immune deficiencies. These medications might cause unwanted side effects. For example, most medications that affect the immune system also trigger the overgrowth of the fungus Candida albicans in the mouth. Other medications can also contribute to loss of the sense of taste and cause foul odors and dry mouth. To lessen the unintended side effects of medication, it is important for seniors to undertake proper oral care.

7—Proper Tooth and Denture Care

Dr. Alisa Kauffman

After lockdown due to COVID-19, I went back into care facilities to provide hands-on care for the residents. What I found was that many of the residents' mouths that we serviced were in awful condition. There are no other words for it. Some residents did not even have toothbrushes in their rooms and could not remember the last time they had their teeth brushed. Plaque and calculus (hard tartar buildup) covered their teeth, and lips were chapped. I even found black mold on one sweet lady's dentures.

Experiencing this broke my heart. It pains me to think that they have been living like this for the past couple of months. Recalling this experience makes me emotional. I surveyed caregivers from facility to facility. They all told me the same thing, "We have anxiety when we are brushing the resident's teeth or removing their dentures."

I believe that this fear comes from the lack of training for caregivers in oral care. And especially during COVID with mask-wearing, oral care is suffering for those who cannot help themselves.

Proper Teeth and Denture Care from the Perspective of Geriatric House Call Dentist

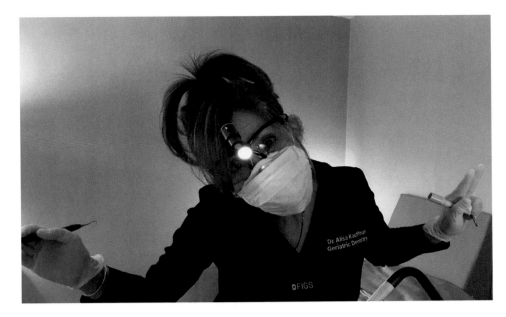

One of the misconceptions that caregivers have is that they should stop brushing the patient's teeth if they see blood. This assumption is wrong. Yes, bleeding gums indicate that the patient has poor oral health and a dental visit is warranted, but do not stop brushing twice a day. Include a gentle alcohol-free oral rinse after brushing. Bleeding gums can also be a dead giveaway that the caregiver is not brushing correctly. It is understandable to be alarmed when blood appears, but what happens to their teeth if the caregiver stops brushing?

Inflammation and redness are common characteristics of patients suffering from poor oral care. Inflammation is the leading cause for the teeth to bleed when the patient's teeth are not brushed or brushed incorrectly. A diagnosis and treatment will be laid out by your dentist, and most likely the first step is a deep cleaning by the dentist or hygienist as soon as possible. An oral rinse should accompany the routine after brushing, and a prescription oral rinse may even be suggested to decrease inflammation and bleeding.

Typically food just sticks or lies on the front of the teeth if it isn't loosened or washed down while drinking water or other liquids with the meal. The food that sticks will eventually cause a white spot, or "initial decay," in dental terms. For weeks or months, this white spot spreads, and the spot deepens, likely causing pain. And if left untreated, the tooth eventually breaks off, leaving the root inside of the gum. I have encountered many patients who suffer from tooth or gum sensitivity stemming from these broken teeth.

Dental providers want to avoid their patients having pain at all costs. When treating the elderly and frail, a dentist trained in geriatrics may elect to use ADA-approved products such as silver diamine fluoride (SDF), proven to keep the decay from progressing. SDF is a liquid applied directly to the initial decay or decay within the tooth to prevent the cavity from progressing or spreading. The silver helps to eradicate the bacteria that cause the decay, and the fluoride component helps the tooth to rebuild, known as remineralization. Unnecessary drilling into the decayed tooth can be avoided with the use of SDF, if the dentist is confident that this is the treatment route appropriate for their patient's individualized needs.

In my practice, drilling on a patient with dementia may be impossible, and SDF is probably my most important product in my practice. It isn't the right treatment choice for everyone, but it's great when you can't drill and fill. This technique as well as the pros and cons should be discussed with the treating dentist.

Seniors are at risk of much more than having bad breath if caregivers and dental professionals fail to care for their teeth. Their gums and teeth can be compromised. It is imperative to brush at the gumline in a light circular motion.

Tools for Proper Mouth, Teeth, and Denture Cleaning

The first tool is the lollipop sponge. It is generally used in hospitals to clean and soothe the patient's mouth and tissues. This tool is not to be used directly on dentures or the patient's teeth due to its ineffectiveness. The sponge is incapable of cleaning plaque off the teeth and should only be used to clean the gums and palate, removing residual food when a toothbrush is not a possibility. Adult toothbrushes are the standard for senior oral care. It is important to choose the most suitable toothbrush. One size does not fit all.

Ensure that the toothbrush has soft bristles, similar to an infant toothbrush. Choosing a toothbrush head with a soft rubber side against the hard plastic is also important because it protects the patient from tooth damage. Too often, seniors lose mouth control or accidentally bite down on the plastic side opposite of the bristles on the toothbrushes, which may cause them to crack or break teeth or fillings. We must be careful with patients who bite while brushing because accidents may happen. The Willo toothbrushing robot was invented to remediate this type of situation.

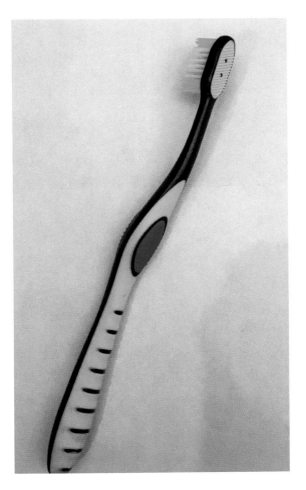

Adult toothbrushes are standard for senior oral health care.

How to Properly Brush Patient's Teeth

Now more than in any era, seniors have teeth for a very long time. It is essential to know how to care for them properly. Caregivers should start by positioning the toothbrush so the first row of bristles is touching below the gumline. There is a small "pocket" between the tooth and gum. This method is best administered when the aide practices this on themselves. The caregiver can practice by taking a toothpick and feeling for that area in their mouth. The area between the teeth and the gums needs to be cleaned effectively using a light circular motion to prevent gingivitis. Gingivitis may progress to the next stage known as periodontitis. Eventually the teeth will become loose, leading to tooth loss.

Automated Brushing

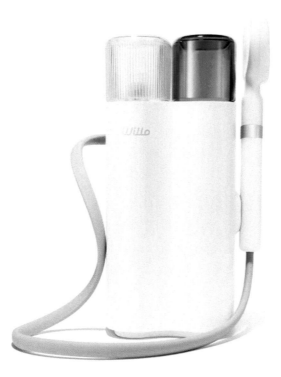

Willo is the first automated oral care robot that gives people of all ages, sizes, and abilities the power to achieve a kinder, more consistent, at-home clean.

Willo was invented to respond to the great need to improve oral health for the disabled population and the patients who need help with their ADLs. Willo is the first automated oral care robot that gives people of all ages, sizes, and abilities the power to achieve a kinder, more consistent, at-home clean. Recognizing this product's transformative nature, Willo decided to target the audience who needs it most, the disabled community.

Willo is the first automated, oral care robot that gives people of all ages, sizes, and abilities the power to achieve a kinder, more consistent, at-home clean. Recognizing the transformative nature of this product, Willo decided to launch first, not just for anyone, but for those who need it most within the differently abled community.

It's so simple to set up and even simpler to use. The magic happens in Willo's comfortable silicone mouthpiece lined with soft bristles that wrap around each arch (all the teeth at the top or all the teeth at the bottom at one time) for a complete clean. While this mouthpiece can benefit anyone, it is an absolute game-changer for caregivers, especially those taking care of patients with dementia. Caregivers are all too familiar with the struggle and concern they have when trying to brush a patient's teeth, but now Willo can take care of the work. Brush positioning, movement, and removal of the rinse mix during a brushing cycle mean caregivers can relax knowing there's no potential for chipping, choking, or discomfort.

Willo, with its automated brushing, spit and foam-free cycle, and chomp-resistant mouthpiece, is poised to empower caregivers and individuals to achieve a more thorough and consistent clean.

See Willo.com for more information. Watch Sonya Dunbar and Dr. Alisa Kauffman demonstrate the Willo robot. Go to our website, TheToothAndNothingButTheTruth.com, the video on Willo.com, as well as all our videos!

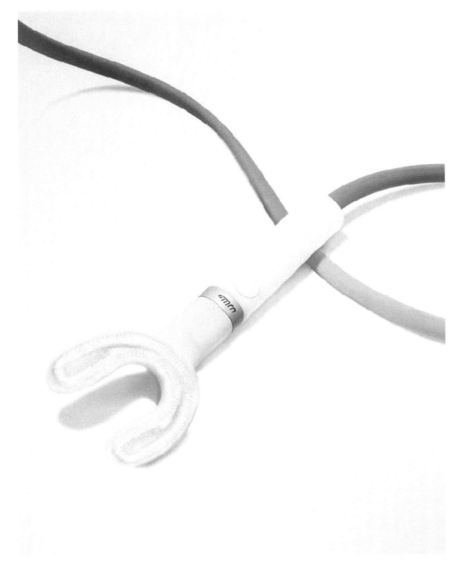

Willo's silicone mouthpiece is lined with soft bristles that wrap around each arch for a complete clean.

Mouthwashes and Fluoride Rinses

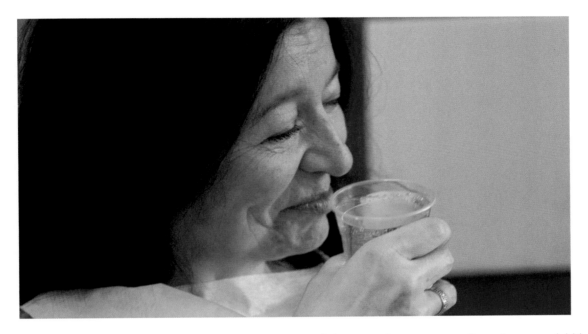

A rinse is recommended to those who can still brush but maybe not as well as they would like.

If an individual can still swish and spit, caregivers are to encourage their patient to use a mouth rinse after brushing. It aids in removing the leftover particles and bacteria that may linger. A fluoride rinse is recommended for those who can still brush but maybe not as well as they would like. This will prevent decay from developing, especially on the front of the teeth where food sticks the most.

I often prescribe a chlorhexidine gluconate rinse for many of my patients who can still effectively swish and spit. This prescribed rinse helps keep the gums infection-free, decreases bleeding, and helps from developing gingivitis/periodontitis. The one side effect is that the teeth may turn a bit grey over time, but the benefit outweighs the risk if it saves the teeth from infection or tooth loss. Please discuss this issue with the dentist, who will help you decide if this treatment works with your treatment plan. I also often recommend an over-the-counter oral rinse that is sulfate-free, pH-balanced, and extremely gentle for those who have sensitive tissues or are prone to apthous ulcers.

Toothpaste Choices

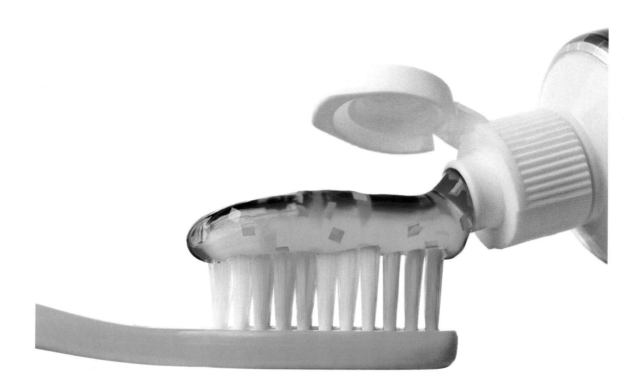

If the patient can swish and spit out excess toothpaste, the toothpaste choice is a personal one.

If the patient can still swish and spit out excess toothpaste, then toothpaste choice is a personal one. I always suggest one that has the fewest amounts of chemicals, has low abrasivity, and are sulfate-free. If they swallow the toothpaste, caregivers will need to be more proactive in choosing one that is not harmful to digest. My solution for those who will swallow toothpaste is to use a xylitol gel. Xylitol is a naturally occurring sugar found in fruits and vegetables and has been found most effective for individuals with dry mouth and those who cannot use traditional toothpaste. The consistency makes it feel like toothpaste and aids in picking up food particles.

How to Care for Edentulous Patients (No Teeth)

Dr. Alisa Kauffman

"Be true to your teeth, and they won't be false to you."
—Soupy Sales

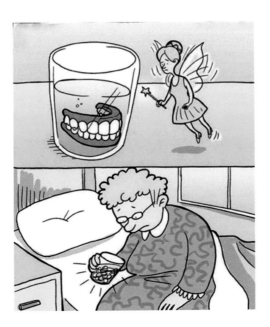

Caregivers must remove and clean the dentures every night and put them away safely in a see-through glass or specified denture case.

f the senior you are caring for wears dentures, the caregiver must remove and clean the dentures every night and put them away safely in a see-through glass or specified denture-only case. Caregivers are reminded that dentures are expensive to replace and difficult to refabricate, especially on a dementia or hospice patient. We don't want to chance that they may be misplaced or lost. That is why putting dentures in their proper cases is vital. Long-term care facility caregivers should avoid storing dentures in anything other than a visible case or one meant only for dentures and encourage residents to do the same. Napkins, tissue, purses, and bags can be thrown away or misplaced. It happens all the time. Losing a patient's dentures compromises the small luxuries seniors hold dear, for instance, eating, chewing, talking, and aesthetics.

This is a difficult subject, but all caregivers should know that it is important to remove the dentures before ever leaving the house by ambulance.

Emergency medical teams and first responders have one job only, to keep the individual in crisis alive. Things happen quickly, and keeping the airway clear is their top priority. This is easier if the patient is not wearing their dentures. Accidents happen, and dentures get misplaced, especially when they do not have permanent IDs placed.

As a caregiver, you must think quickly and remove the dentures before leaving the house! I am telling you this so you will be well-prepared. I hope this scenario never occurs, but if it does, please remove the dentures in their mouth. You can always bring the dentures to them later after they are settled in the hospital or place them back in their mouths when they return home.

This is a very important message to repeat so please remember. Remove all partial or complete dentures if you need to be transported in an emergency, even if it means posting a reminder note on the door for all to see.

Denture Removal

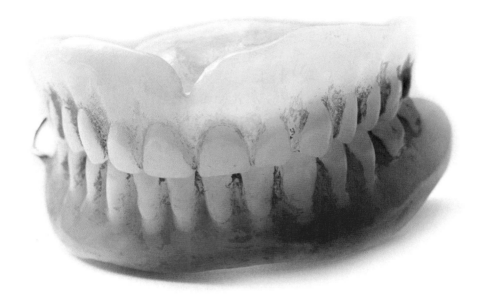

If caregivers do not remove dentures every night, the tissue in the mouth
can grow around the denture, causing tissue overgrowth.

In care facilities, denture removal and cleaning are extremely necessary to the daily routine. It is rare to hear caregivers talking or educating others about it. Removing and cleaning dentures is not a walk in the park. However, it is necessary for caregivers to truly master this chore. Most dentures are removed by placing your index finger between the denture and the gumline midway back on the cheek side. Pull it down quickly if it is a top denture or pull it up quickly if it is a bottom denture. Sometimes the patient may need a denture adhesive, making it a bit more challenging to remove. Nevertheless, do not despair. It will come out.

There may be some resistance, but if you know that the patient has dentures, never stop trying to get them out. I cannot tell you how many times caregivers are fooled and do not realize that their patient wears dentures. It's imperative to know as a caregiver if you will be doing oral care on teeth or dentures. I get a call every now and then that a patient is complaining of pain, and that pain is from dentures that have not been removed for ages! No one knew they were dentures and not their real teeth!

As a caregiver, the consequence of not removing the dentures every night is the eventual possibility that the tissue in the mouth can grow around the denture, causing tissue overgrowth (dentally known as hyperplasia of the tissues), causing an infection and/or swelling that causes much pain. Sometimes the patient will be forced to stop wearing the denture, and this unfortunate event will change their quality of life. The denture can usually be adjusted away from the irritated area; however, dentures should only be adjusted as a last resort. So remember to remove the complete or partial dentures at night and let the mouth and tissues rest.

Caregivers should also be reminded that dentures are fragile as they are made of a select type of plastic. Always carefully clean them in a sink filled with water to avoid dropping them. They can fracture and may even break in half. Should that occur, it is necessary to call a dentist to repair them. Denture repair is not a quick YouTube fix. Dentures must be repaired only by professionally trained laboratory technicians. Buying a self-repair kit sold online or at the local pharmacy will most likely render the already broken dentures unrepairable. Please heed my warning! Call your dentist. Usually it's a quick and affordable repair.

Partial Dentures versus Complete Dentures

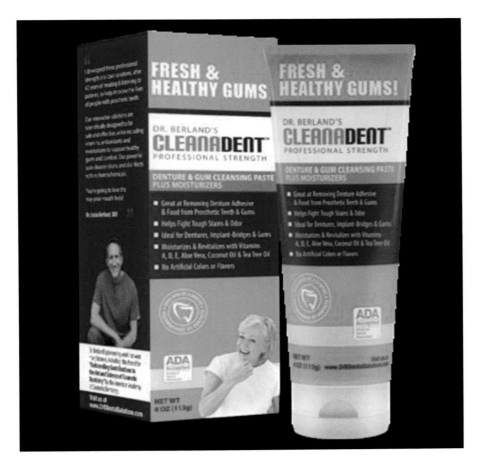

To clean partial dentures, remove and clean them using Dr. Berlard's Cleanadent Paste.

Wearing a complete denture means that you are completely edentulous (no teeth remaining in the mouth) and a prosthesis replaces all your teeth. Partial dentures replace one or more missing teeth by anchoring onto the remaining natural teeth. To clean them, remove the partial dentures and brush both the partial and remaining real teeth, which remain in the mouth.

I only recommend Dr. Berland's Cleanadent (drbsolutions.com), the only product I know of on the market that is ADA-approved that can be used on both your natural teeth as well as on the denture teeth and denture as a whole. Remove the denture by using your thumb or index finger under the clasp and pull down if it is an upper partial or under the clasp and pull up for a lower partial.

There are three types of partial dentures you may see as a caregiver. And again, some people may fool you. I never knew my grandmother had a partial denture until she got sick, and only then did I notice it in a glass in her bathroom.

The first type of partial denture has a predominantly metal frame. Patients generally find this to have the best fit. Clean it by brushing it everywhere with Dr. Berland's Denture & Mouth Toothbrush and disinfect it in the Liquid Crystals by drbsolutions.com and water for up to fifteen minutes. If you do not remove the partial denture while brushing the remaining teeth, food and bacteria will collect around and under the clasps that hold it on their real teeth. This will eventually lead to decay and possible tooth loss.

I get the occasional call that the patient's partial denture is loose and no longer fits. I usually go intending to tighten a loose clasp but unfortunately find the clasped tooth decayed and broken off to the gumline. The broken tooth must then be extracted, and a new clasp must be added to a different, healthy tooth. It is a complicated procedure and must be sent to the laboratory for repair.

The second type of denture is a soft, flexible partial denture that is popular when deciding which partial denture offers is the best fit. There is no metal. The clasps can be clear, pink, or even tooth-colored. This type of partial denture looks very natural in the mouth. Because it is soft and flexible, it can be kinder to the tissues and easier to get used to. But this type of partial denture is more porous, and that attracts more food and bacteria.

Like all dentures, these must be removed at night and if the individual cooperates after every meal. Soak it for fifteen minutes in cool water and Liquid Crystals by Dr. B. Then leave it clean in a case or clear glass overnight.

If you step on it or accidentally put it in the washing machine, it is not repairable. So please be careful. If a natural tooth breaks, you may not be able to add a new clasp to a flexible partial denture. That is an important consideration when deciding which partial denture is right for a patient with dementia. For these patients, I always recommend a metal partial or an all-acrylic partial because it is easier to repair and adjust. This should be discussed with your dentist at the treatment planning visit.

The third type of partial denture is an all-acrylic (all-plastic) partial with wire clasps. Like a complete denture, it is repairable, and you can easily add a new wire clasp if needed. It can also be converted to a full denture if all the teeth require removal in the future.

This partial denture is also referred to as a flipper because they flip in and out. They can replace one or several teeth by attaching to the remaining teeth. Of course, these also need to be removed at night. All clasps are food traps that can eventually cause decay.

My only word of warning is to be careful when the flipper is small enough that it can be swallowed if accidentally dislodged. If the patient has dementia, you need to think carefully about the repercussions if you can't find it in the mouth. This type of partial must be monitored and removed every night. It should be permanently removed if there is even the slightest possibility of swallowing it.

If you are caring for an individual in a long-term care or assisted-living facility, my best advice is to have the patient's name or ID placed in the patient's partial or full denture. If a lost denture is found, they can easily identify the rightful owner.

I have worked in many nursing homes and assisted-living facilities over the years, and identifying a found denture is a lost cause. A denture lab can easily place a name or ID number into the denture. If the care facility does not provide that service, take them to your own personal dentist to get this done.

What You Should Do If the Denture Becomes Loose and Slips When Eating?

Over time, the bone, tissues, and fat in the mouth change. It is even more common if there is a recent weight loss. Gum tissue naturally shrinks, bone wears away, and the denture will become less stable and more uncomfortable. When this happens, there are four treatment options. The patient, family, caregiver, and dentist determine the final decision.

Denture Adhesive

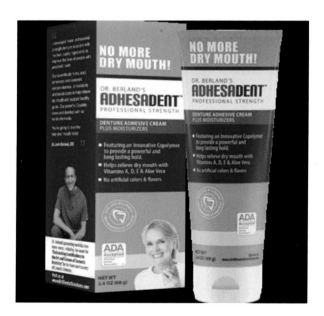

I always give my patients a full-sized tube of Dr. Berland's Adhesadent ™(drbsolutions.com) since it has the most powerful hold and moisturizes gums unlike other brands of adhesive.

It is the only denture adhesive that helps relieve dry mouth with vitamins A, D, and E as well as aloe vera. Adhesadent does not contain any artificial flavors, colors, or zinc. And Adhesadent is the first and only denture adhesive developed by a dentist to earn the American Dental Association Seal of Acceptance. This is important to me, as the feedback I get from my patients is that it is the best brand on the market.

Soft Denture Reline

An experienced dentist can usually provide a soft reline in one visit. With proper care, a soft reline may function for six months to two years. Because it is soft, many people find soft relines very comfortable. Remember to clean the inside of the denture gently so the soft reline does not get dislodged and only soak it in the Liquid Crystals for three to five minutes to kill the bacteria that accumulate over twelve hours. It should be kept overnight in warm water only so the reline remains in place.

Hard Denture Reline

On the tissue side, a hard denture reline is similar to a new denture. Proper fitting may require additional adjustments. A hard denture reline may be accomplished chairside in one visit, but it is usually best finished in the dental laboratory. This requires the patient to be without the denture for a few days to finish.

A New Denture

Depending on the person and their health and weight fluctuations, a denture should be replaced at least every five to ten years. Most dentures are kept way past their expiration date. Most often, the best treatment is a new denture. However, new dentures are not always possible for people with Alzheimer's disease, dementia, or any neurodegenerative disease. For these individuals, a soft or hard reline may be the only option.

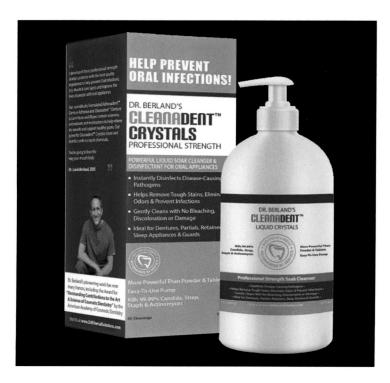

Soak your dentures in Dr. Berland's Cleanadent™ Liquid Crystals for at least fifteen minutes.

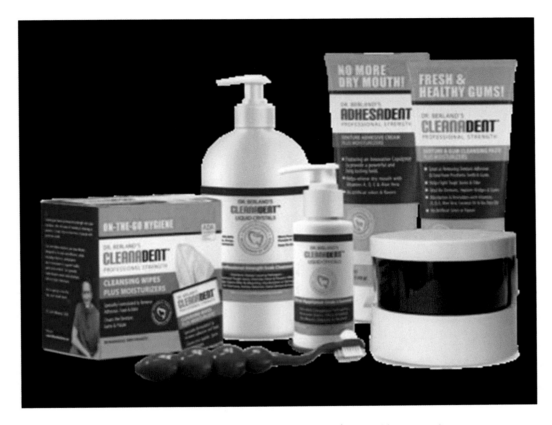

Dr. Berland's Cleanadent Denture Solution Kit contains
ingredients that we can recognize and pronounce.

Summary

Brush the patient's teeth and dentures at least twice a day. Caregivers should especially brush the patient's teeth at night. At night there is a considerable buildup of collected food and a full day's worth of bacteria. Use a soft toothbrush and a fluoride toothpaste, such as those in Dr. Berland's Denture Care System. This practice should be followed up by a gentle mouth rinse. If a full or partial denture is worn, caregivers must remove it, soak it, and leave it in a clear glass or denture container with a cleanser like Dr. Berland's Cleanadent's Crystals.

The denture should never be stored in tissue or anything other than a proper denture container. If the dentures feel loose while speaking or eating, try a denture adhesive such as Dr. Berland's Adhesadent. If that isn't sufficient, call your dentist as a reline or new denture may be necessary. Caregivers should never attempt to repair a broken denture but call a professional instead. Dentures should have IDs placed so they are easily returned should they become misplaced, especially in long-term care facilities. And never wear your dentures if you must go in an ambulance or to the hospital. Bring them later when you are settled in your room.

Sonya and I recommend Dr. Berland's Denture Care System with ingredients that we can recognize and pronounce. The Liquid Crystal™ disinfecting soak cleanser is easy to use. It kills dangerous pathogens, such as Candida Albicans, Streptococcus, Staphylococcus, Actinomyces, and E. Coli. We like to use the product by simply soaking the dentures for ten minutes in water and four Liquid Crystal pumps. After soaking the dentures, caregivers should rinse the dentures under cool running water. If there is a soft reline, they should soak them in cool water and the Liquid Crystal for no more than fifteen minutes to preserve the soft liner's integrity.

Using the Liquid Crystal in a Sonic Cleaner will improve efficiency. We also recommend Dr. B.'s Denture & Mouth Toothbrush and Cleanadent Paste™ to clean and remove biofilm from the denture and the gums, tongue, cheeks, palate, and any remaining teeth. If the denture has an inside reline, caregivers must brush very gently not to dislodge the reline material away from the denture. Cleanadent Wipes™ can also be used to clean the inside of relines. They are convenient for cleaning both the mouth and the denture while reducing gagging. Caregivers should refrain from using regular toothpaste on dentures because it will cause microscopic scratches that collect stain, odor, bacteria, and fungi colonization.

Watch Sonya Dunbar and Dr. Alisa Kauffman discuss Dr. Berland's denture care products. Go to our website, TheToothAndNothingButTheTruth.com, to view this video on Dr. B. Dental Solutions and all our videos!

8—Hospice Care

Dr. Alisa Kauffman

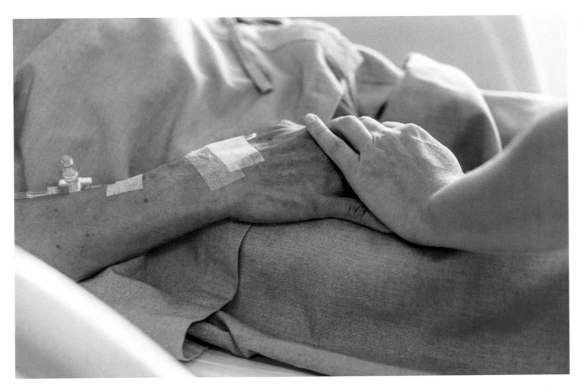

While in hospice care, the caregivers' number-one focus is to provide compassionate care for patients.

Hospice care focuses specifically on patients' daily quality of life for those experiencing chronic and fatal illnesses. While in hospice care, the caregivers' number-one focus is to provide compassionate care for patients. The patient needs to live as comfortably as possible without the cause of any additional discomfort.

I often think about my patient Helen who was in hospice care for three years. Yes, I thought hospice care was always short and always with the same unfortunate ending. But that wasn't the case with Helen. She was alert and had a great attitude. She insisted that the nursing home continue making dental appointments with me. She knew that she might not finish her dental work, but heck, life wasn't getting in her way. Helen told me that she wanted to look pretty when she met Jesus and when she reunited with her family and friends. Helen lived through the dental work for about three more years in hospice care with her new teeth and smile. I often think about her infectious attitude, smile, and bravery.

How to Meet the Oral Care Needs of Those in Hospice Care

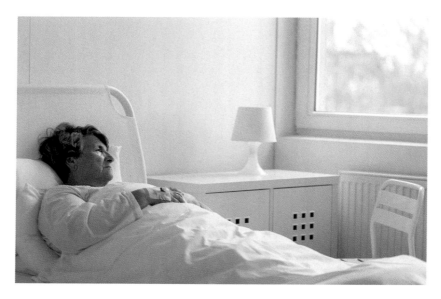

When treating a hospice patient, we must only address the tooth or teeth in question. Non-mandatory dental work is prohibited at this stage, unless the patient requests it and the family agrees.

Dentists and dental hygienists are instrumental in hospice care. Oral care professionals need to monitor patients' mouths for broken or loose teeth, possibly causing them unnecessary pain. Our duty as caregivers and oral health professionals is to maintain good patient hygiene, to ensure health and wellness.

Palliative care for those in hospice should include cleaning the patients' dentures and making sure they fit well. Teeth should also be brushed and the mouth kept moist. Xerostomia, or dry mouth, is painful. Keep the mouth moisturized by using water and moisturizing products. Trauma, such as biting or sucking the lip and grinding of the teeth, must be addressed, and a biting or grinding guard must be fabricated if possible.

If an intraoral examination reveals a tumor or a fungal infection, it must be diagnosed and also treated if possible.

Hospice patients call for close observation. Caregivers must always inform us of any changes in the patient's eating habits. Holding the side of the face may indicate tooth pain or irritation. Any redness or swelling on the face should be immediately addressed. It is not uncommon for elders in hospice to be uncommunicative or even in a coma-like state. Since it may be impossible for the patient to communicate in any way, the caregiver must be intuitive to their needs. It is up to the caregiver or hospice nurse or physician to call a dentist if changes that could be tooth related occur.

When treating a hospice patient, we must only address the tooth or teeth in question. Non-mandatory dental work is prohibited at this stage unless the patient requests it and the family agrees. The issues that call for immediate treatment are as follows:

- If there are teeth causing pain or are loose or if there are any areas of swelling, though it may be extensive, antibiotic therapy or extraction would be necessary.

- Trauma such as biting or sucking the lip, grinding of the teeth, or sharp teeth that may cut the tongue or lip may warrant a custom plastic guard or a simple smoothing of the teeth involved.

- If an intraoral examination reveals a fungal or bacterial infection, a prescribed treatment would be recommended.

- If the denture is causing pain and the tissues demonstrate trauma, it should be adjusted or even permanently removed.

- A broken denture should be repaired as quickly as possible.

Despite our quest for pain-free living, these health concerns can intensify fatality and pain.

Summary

Oral care for the hospice patient should always focus on maintaining the usual daily routine. Caregivers are responsible for monitoring for any changes in a patient's eating habits, redness of the face, or swelling. These details are telltale signs of dental issues and oral pain. Remember that the goal is to ensure that we provide the best remaining quality of life for patients.

9—House Call Dentistry

Dr. Alisa Kauffman

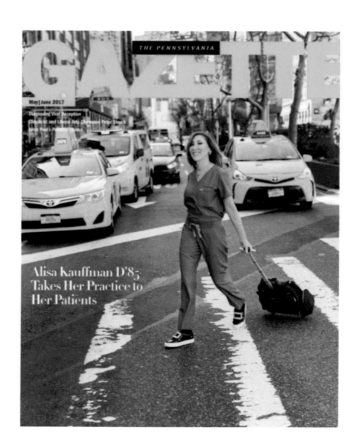

n 1988, I had an epiphany. My best friend's father had impeccable oral health. He knew the importance of great oral hygiene and was on a regular every-three-month schedule with his hygienist. However, a stroke left him without speech and the ability to brush and floss his teeth independently.

When it came time to see the hygienist after his stroke, he had to cancel. That was my moment to step in and assist him. I obtained his most recent x-rays, assembled a mobile kit, and cleaned his teeth as he laid comfortably in bed. It became a regular thing for us. He was the first patient I attended to in their home. Traveling to people's homes in New York City has changed my definition of owning a dental practice. I never knew that practice ownership could be so flexible for patients.

Characteristics of a House Call Dentist

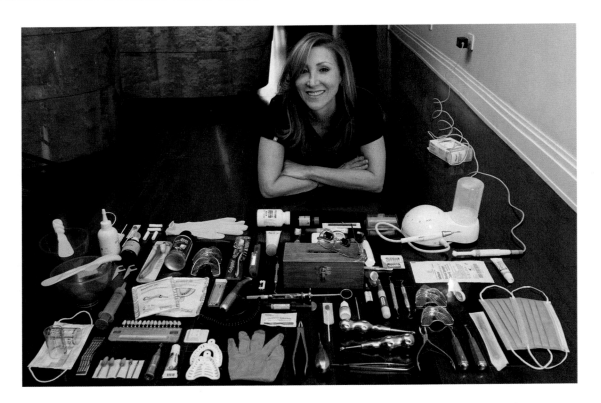

House call dentistry is necessary for aging patients who need to be treated in their homes because they are unable to get to a traditional dental office. The most important consideration in this industry is access. Under the umbrella of access, it is essential to focus on obtaining care for the patient, working with the patient's mobility, and maintaining effective communication between the dental professionals and caregivers.

GeriatricHouseCallDentistry.com is a necessary service for those who are homebound or on hospice. Everyone deserves to have a dentist in their area who is willing to help. There are many expectations when trusting someone in the comfort of their apartment or home, from being proficient and professional to friendly and comforting. A geriatric house call dentist must be a trained professional who feels confident and comfortable working on this growing population of fragile adults, those who also deserve the highest caliber of dental treatment. Most importantly, they must have a passion for being a part of patient healing. I truly love helping this underserved group, whether I am extracting a painful tooth or seeing patients take their first bite of food with the custom, well-fitted dentures that I created.

What to Expect on the First-Time Visit

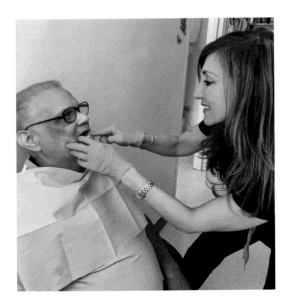

Home call dental services have quickly become one of the most unmet areas of need within geriatric health care because of increased life expectancy due to various medical advances. The health-care world has seen an increase in the market to identify and effectively service unique geriatric needs. Websites such as CaringAndAble.com help to identify products and services that caregivers may be looking for, from effective and safe oral care products to geriatric care management and dentists or hygienists who can treat patients in their homes. Geriatric dental care has resulted in a movement of homebound geriatric dentists providing service for the immobile elders. There is a large gap between the amount of elderly who need homebound dental care and the health-care workforce available to provide it.

Expect the first dental visit to address the emergency need as well as create a treatment plan for future visits. If there is no emergency, a first visit will include a comprehensive exam on the teeth, gums, tongue, and tissues. There will also be an oral cancer exam and an extraoral exam of the face and neck. X-rays may or may not be taken, and a generalized prophy may be done. If more treatment is necessary, the treatment plan should be in writing so those who make the decisions can decide the best next steps.

Geriatric Knowledge and Professionalism

When it comes to dentistry, there is a world of difference between treating a toddler with her first tooth and treating an elder patient with missing teeth. The dental issues that elders experience are unique. Some problems involve broken painful teeth or dentures that no longer fit well. Dentists trained in geriatrics will also address the psychological implications that have developed because of these discomforts.

Although the practice is done at home, standards for cleanliness and sanitation should never be compromised. Disposable instruments and single-use products are used when possible, and others are sterilized in an autoclave before use. Correct protective gear must be worn by the dentist, including strict handwashing and gloves.

Dental professionals have to be fully informed about common health conditions affecting their elderly patients and the medications that accompany those conditions. Often medications are prescribed before a dentist can even treat the patients. And sometimes medications such as blood thinners may need to be held for a few days before any dental treatment can be done. Your house call dentist must have the list of all medications, including vitamins, before the first visit to avoid the risk of possible side effects or complications and should be in contact with the primary care physician, nurse practitioner, or physician's assistant to discuss any concerns before starting any treatment.

Flexibility

Providing dental treatment in the home can be challenging. Some patients will only be comfortable sitting in a specific chair, and others must lay flat in the bed to be treated. The actual working space may be tight and inconvenient, making movement and accessibility a challenge. The bed may need to be moved or the rails on the side of the bed temporarily lowered.

The caregiver should also be prepared to make some space for the dentist's equipment and supplies before they arrive. Bright lights worn on the dentist's eye loops are usually worn for perfect field vision, but extra light or lamps in the room are always appreciated.

Some patients may present problems behaviorally if they have conditions such as dementia, Alzheimer's disease, or Lewy body dementia. Geriatric house call dentists must be flexible at all times. A house call dentist must be willing to work around the patient's treatment preferences and be equipped to handle unusual family requests as well. Most importantly, patients must be treated wherever they feel the most comfortable. Being treated in the comfort of their home environment with faces they recognize make the treatment they receive more relaxed and stress-free.

Compassion and Cost

Perhaps the most essential aspect of geriatric house call dentistry is compassion. Dental professionals who genuinely have a heart for elders change lives. Compassion for this profession ensures patience, perseverance, and commitment with a heart for aging adults and a love for dentistry. A geriatric house call dentist must come prepared with a smile and a skillful hand. A welcoming smile instantly brings calm and comfort to her patients.

The cost of a geriatric house call visit will vary by the city, state, and provider. Some providers accept insurance while others don't. Just remember that this is quite different from a brick-and-mortar office. The dentist may only be able to see three to six patients a day as opposed to eight to ten patients. The dentist will need to be compensated for giving you the necessary time for completing the service, which normally takes thirty to seventy-five minutes to accommodate the physical or mental challenges involved. We can only hope that federally funded programs in the future will recognize this type of service as necessary and will fall under the umbrella of insured care.

Open-Door Policy

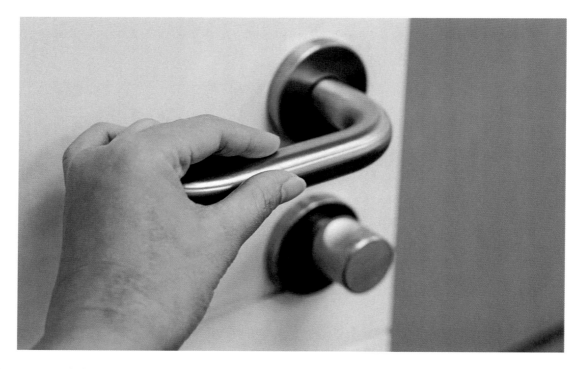

While I do not have a building with an actual open door, I will emphasize being readily available for my patients and their family members.

While I do not have an office building with an actual open door, I emphasize being readily available for my patients and their family members. My direct phone number is always available. I strive to answer whenever possible or return the call quickly. Families expect that an emergency needs to be addressed immediately. Open communication concerning questions and concerns is valued and encouraged. A complete medical history form must be completed, and old x-rays are extremely valuable for those who may not be able to cooperate in taking new ones. Clear photographs taken with a smartphone of the situation help assess if this is a true emergency. The dentist and caregiver together decide if this is an emergency situation or one that can wait. The dentist should also have access to the primary care physician's number because we believe that systemic health and oral health are directly linked. And we must coordinate our treatments and philosophies while sharing this patient.

10—The Many Types of Mobile Dentistry

Sonya Dunbar, the Geriatric Toothfairy

Let's explore the different types.

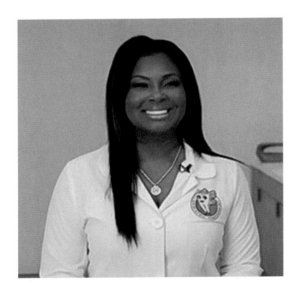

added this chapter to the book because access to care is essential and so many do not get the necessary care they need. Many underserved and minority communities suffer needlessly because of lack of dental care. Mobile dentistry allows the dental professional to take dentistry to patients who might not or cannot come to you.

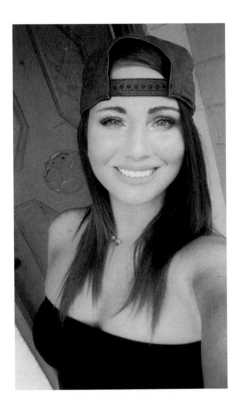

I dedicate this chapter to Brittany, a beautiful young lady who lost her life to fentanyl poisoning. Growing up, Brittany was a light to all who met her. When she was about five years old, her mother would sing to her at bedtime. One of her favorite songs was "You Are My Sunshine."

One night, Brittany stopped her mother mid-verse and said, "Mommy, I'm not your sunshine. I am your Daughtershine!"

And that she was. Her loving spirit and radiant smile were light to all who knew her. She joined her mother as a hygiene assistant after graduating from high school. She remained in the dental field until her passing. She loved to make others smile.

Just before her twenty-second birthday, Brittany suffered a devastating knee injury while attending a concert. Another concertgoer fell backward into the side of her right knee and tore the ACL from the bone. She underwent an ACL replacement surgery and was prescribed prescription opioids for her recovery. Unfortunately the surgery was not a success. Brittany continued to experience pain and instability months beyond when she should have recovered fully.

Eight months of pain and prescriptions later, a second ACL replacement was performed. While her rehabilitation from the second surgery was successful, Brittany realized that she was addicted to the pain medication prescribed to her for the previous eight months. That rehabilitation would become a fight for her very life.

When the prescriptions were no longer available, Brittany turned to illicit means to keep her from being "dope sick." At a street cost of $40 per pill, she would sometimes spend her entire paycheck before she got it, just to make it through the week. Her prescription opioid addiction turned to heroin addiction, and things spiraled out of control. Thankfully, Brittany had the full support of her family and finally entered inpatient treatment in March 2018.

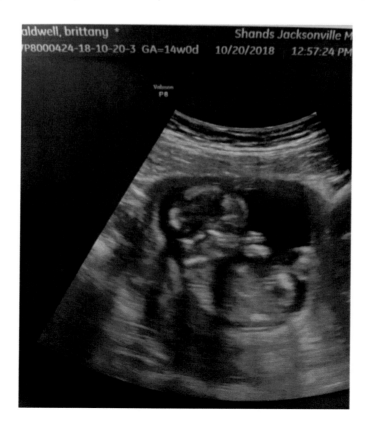

Three months later, Brittany was back! She was glowing again and not just because she was sober and healthy. Brittany was pregnant with her first child. She was so excited. She had always been great with children, and she was thrilled to become a mother. She was pretty nauseous in the beginning, but it progressively got worse throughout the pregnancy. She was diagnosed with hyperemesis gravida, a severe form of morning sickness. She discontinued all of her medication for addiction, depression, and anxiety that she had been prescribed in rehab. She couldn't keep anything down anyway.

In late October 2018, Brittany's maternal grandfather was hospitalized with end-stage COPD and lung cancer. She spent many hours with her mother at his bedside and prayed that he would be able to come home for Thanksgiving. It was their favorite holiday, and she was so proud to be carrying his first great-grandchild. Boy or girl, her child would be called Ryatt. She coaxed her grandfather into getting well soon because he would be a great-grandfather soon. She was already halfway through her pregnancy. It was not to be. She spent Thanksgiving night and most of the next day at her grandfather's bedside. He had just been moved to rehab, but he was suddenly in a lot of pain. She shared Thanksgiving leftovers with her parents. Her mother dropped her off at her paternal grandmother's house, where she was living.

As her mother was signing her grandfather into emergency surgery for a perforated bowel the following day, she received the call that Brittany had relapsed and that she and Ryatt were gone. Her grandfather made it through surgery but passed eight days later, joining his granddaughter and great-granddaughter for eternity.

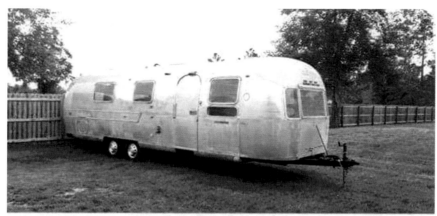

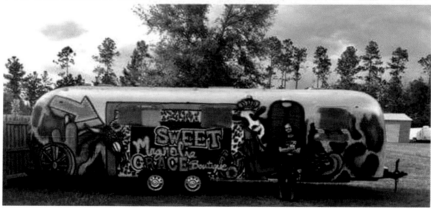

The COVID pandemic of 2020 pales in comparison to the opioid pandemic. Both are ravaging our country for more than a decade now. It is slowly but surely taking an entire generation of our children. It does not discriminate and shows no mercy. Brittany's mother, Cami Caldwell, hopes to change that in any way she can by providing understanding, support, and, most importantly, resources to those struggling to get and stay sober.

Cami Caldwell is a licensed dental hygienist entering twenty-four years of practice in Florida. She has founded a 501(c)(3) nonprofit organization in loving memory of her daughter and granddaughter, Daughtershine, Inc. It is a mobile dentistry clinic whose mission is to provide free dental care to those in recovery in Northeast Florida, to erase the stigma associated with addiction and dental disease and to encourage recovery one smile at a time.

Mobile Dentistry

Mobile dentistry involves dental professionals, like dentists, dental hygienists, and dental assistants traveling in vans with their equipment to provide care in patients' homes.[21] This increases access to oral care to vulnerable populations and reduces dental pain. As such, mobile dentistry is greatly beneficial to organizations, schools, and the community. There is demand for mobile dentistry in different areas, including geriatric, school base, special needs, corporate, addiction recovery facilities, homebound, whitening, and mobile dentistry. These faces of mobile dentistry are discussed.

Addiction Recovery Facilities

According to the Centers for Disease Control and Prevention (CDC), 11.2 percent of Americans who are twelve years and over reported use of a type of illicit substance in 2017.[23] People addicted to illicit substances spend a lot of time intoxicated or trying to obtain drugs, at the expense of oral care, such as brushing their teeth or visiting the dentist.[24] Poor oral hygiene increases their risk of oral complications. For example, many heroin addicts suffer from tooth decay and missing teeth due to malnutrition and poor oral care.[25] People who abuse marijuana are also likely to suffer from oral complications, such as acidic erosion of tooth enamel.

While the oral treatment needs of people recovering from addiction are high, a large population of them do not receive oral care due to challenges, such as poor collaboration between dental professionals and other health-care providers serving addicts and lack of knowledge on how to treat drug addicts.[26] Lack of dental treatment makes it difficult for recovering addicts to eat and may damage their self-esteem, making their emotional recovery difficult.[27] A dental van visiting an addiction recovery facility increases the access to oral care to recovering addicts, which will rebuild their self-esteem and aid emotional recovery.

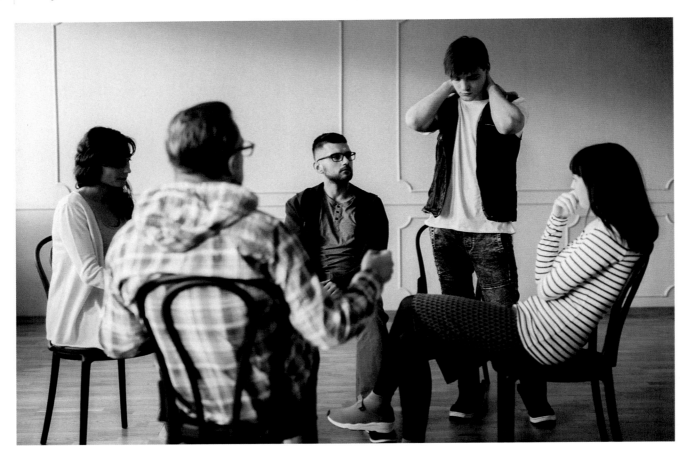

Lack of dental treatment makes it difficult for recovering addicts to eat and may damage their self-esteem, making their emotional recovery difficult.

Geriatric Mobile Dentistry

Sonya Dunbar, the Geriatric Toothfairy

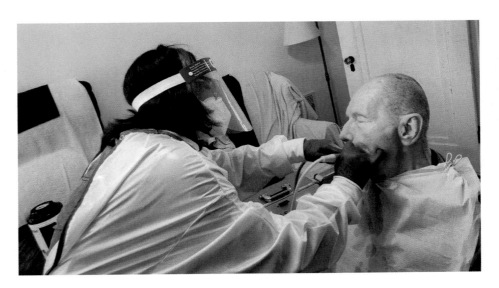
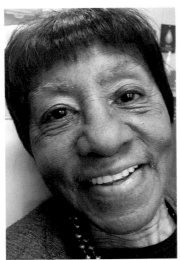

M obile dentistry meets people who will never walk through your office door but will allow you to walk through theirs. As Americans live longer, the number of seniors continues to increase. By 2060, 98 million people in America will be aged sixty-five years and older.[28] Older adults are more vulnerable to oral diseases as they rely on others to meet their oral care needs. The seniors themselves might also not be motivated to clean their teeth, especially if they have to attend to other pressing health issues.[29] This causes bacteria to accumulate in their mouths, leading to infection and periodontal disease.[30] Periodontal disease increases the vulnerability of older adults to aspiration pneumonia,[31] the leading cause of death from infection in adults aged sixty-five years and older, accounting for 13 to 48 percent of infection in nursing homes.[32]

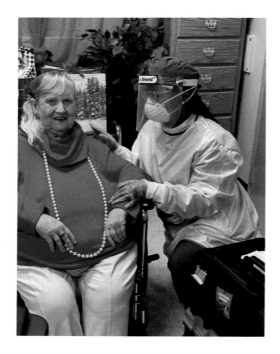

The services of geriatric mobile dentists would greatly benefit seniors living in long-term care facilities.

Studies also link poor oral care to other causes of death of seniors, including cardiovascular disease,[33] cancer,[34] and respiratory disease. [35] Other diseases linked to poor oral care are Alzheimer's,[35] dementia,[37] and involuntary weight loss.[38]

Therefore, the services of geriatric mobile dentists would greatly benefit seniors living in long-term care facilities. The dental vans have a chair for seniors who walk or use walkers to sit on during examinations and another for the professional. The dental professionals also have a bag with equipment they might need, such as a camera and light. They conduct comprehensive exams and x-rays, clean dentures, fix partials, and perform fillings and extractions.

During these exams, dental professionals can detect some diseases, such as oral cancer, and refer the patient to an oncologist for treatment. In extreme weather conditions, the dental professionals offer care inside the facilities where seniors are most comfortable. Most of the facilities do not have a place for a dental office, so they have to improvise. This might entail treating the patients in any private space that they can sterilize and set up their equipment, including bathrooms, shower rooms, and back of hallways. Some residents are confined to their beds or comatose, and the professionals might need to offer care besides their bed. Others seniors could also be on a Geri chair, or a wheelchair, and they might have to bend to attend to them.

Setup: Mobile Dentistry

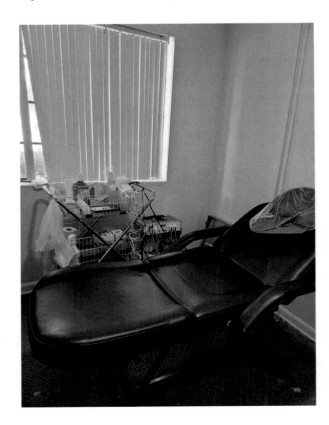 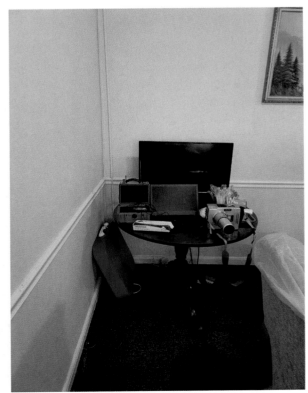

Special Needs Mobile Dentistry

One out of five children in the United States has a special health-care need.[39] Children and youth with special health care needs have different physical, emotional, behavioral, and developmental differences from their peers and may need more care.[40] Others may also have constant medical needs.

Studies show that people with developmental disabilities, like cerebral palsy, Down syndrome, and autism, are more likely to suffer from oral health problems such as gum disease, tooth decay, malocclusion, damaging oral habits, delayed tooth eruption, as well as trauma and injury from accidents.[41] Children with special health-care needs also find it more difficult to access dental care.[42] The situation is worse for special needs children with severe needs, teenagers, or those who live in areas with a shortage of health-care professionals.

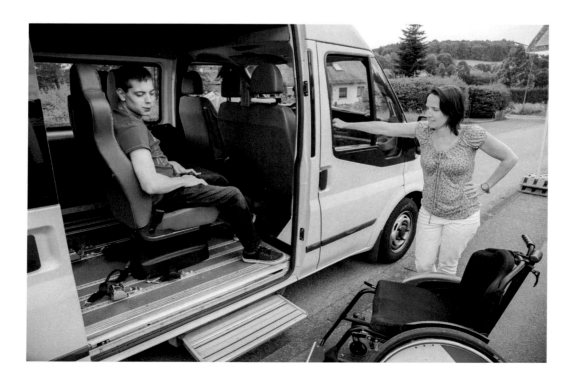

People with special needs may find it difficult to get to the dentist.

Mobile dentistry would increase access to dental care to this vulnerable group. Dental vans park outside the homes of special needs patients, who then leave their homes and get into the vans to receive dental care. The units are spacious enough for someone who is in a wheelchair and contain other useful equipment, like restraints. Sometimes the dental professionals take their gear inside the home to provide treatment. When dental professionals offer care in an environment that is familiar to patients, they are less likely to be anxious.[43]

Corporate Mobile Dentistry

Mobile dentistry has traditionally been used to narrow the access gap for people who have transportation challenges, such as children and seniors. However, it is increasingly valuable to corporations. A study by the American Dental Association shows that over half of adults who have private dental insurance have not seen a dentist for over a year.[44] Other workers are hesitant to go to the dentist because they do not want to miss work. A mobile dentist will make it easier for employees to access oral care and use their insurance coverage since the dental van parks outside the office. The dental professionals offer employees dental treatment, such as fillings, composites, cleanings, or root canals during their lunch break. This reduces the number of days people miss work and increases productivity. Dental professionals can also catch dental problems early and help reduce emergency room visits.

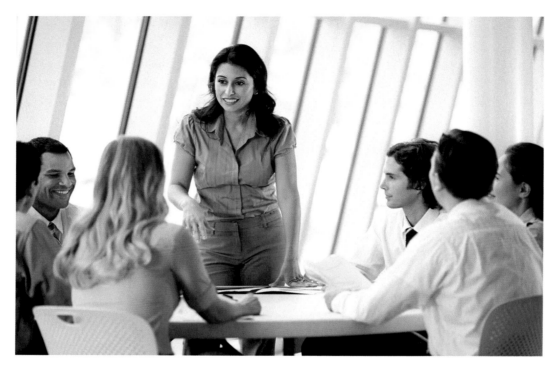

Employees do not see the dentist because they do not want to take time off work.

Homebound Mobile Dentistry

Homebound populations consist of non-institutionalized groups of people who are unable to leave their homes because of physical, psychiatric, or social constraints.[45] Many of them include women and people who suffer from chronic diseases, such as obesity, diabetes, MS, and hypertension. [46] While homebound patients are interested in receiving oral treatment, it is difficult for them to access it due to health and transportation barriers.[47] Mobile dentistry would make dental care more accessible to homebound patients as the dental van parks outside their homes and the patients can walk into it to receive treatment. If the patient is unable or unwilling to leave their home, the dental professional can bring their equipment into the patient's home and treat them from there.

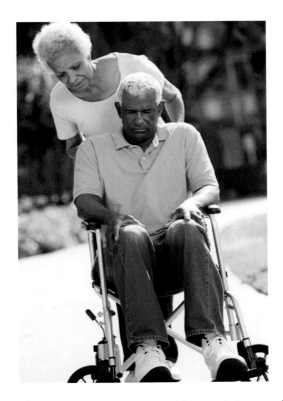

While homebound patients are interested in receiving oral treatment, it is difficult for them to access it due to health and transportation barriers.

Whitening Mobile Dentistry

Ninety-nine percent of Americans believe that a smile is an important asset and have an aversion to discolored, stained, or yellow teeth.[48] Hence, tooth whitening is one of the most commonly requested dental procedures.[49] Tooth whitening is an effective way of lightening the color of the teeth without removing its surface. Teeth get discolored by coffee, tea, smoking cigarettes, or wine. Other causes of tooth discoloration are age or using certain medications. People whiten discolored teeth in different ways, but the most common tooth whitening procedures are supervised tooth bleaching done at home or in a dentist's office.[50]

As the demand for tooth whitening grows, the opportunity for mobile dentists to exploit this need also increases. The dental vans can visit people's homes, offices, bridal showers, bachelorette parties, and teeth whitening parties to offer tooth whitening services. To start a mobile tooth whitening dentistry, you might need a booth, salon, or vehicle and supplies.

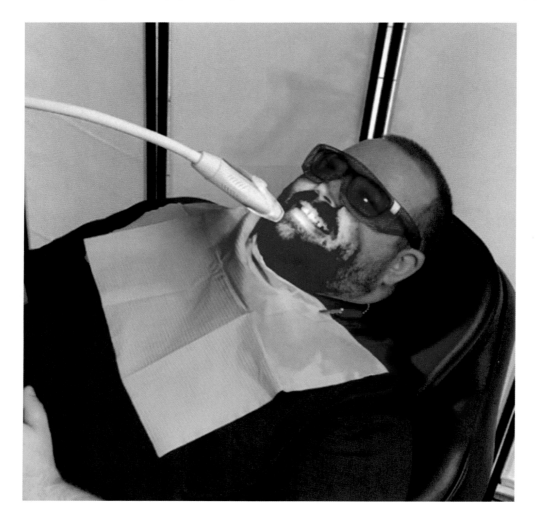

Mobile dental professionals can venture into tooth whitening,
the most common requested dental procedure.

Cost Differences Between Mobile Dentistry and a Brick-and-Mortar Dentist's Office

Whether you want to open a brick-and-mortar dentist office or run a mobile practice, you will need start-up capital. However, the equipment you need to set up a mobile dentistry is not as expensive as what you would buy when setting up a stationary dentist's office.

The following table shows the differences.

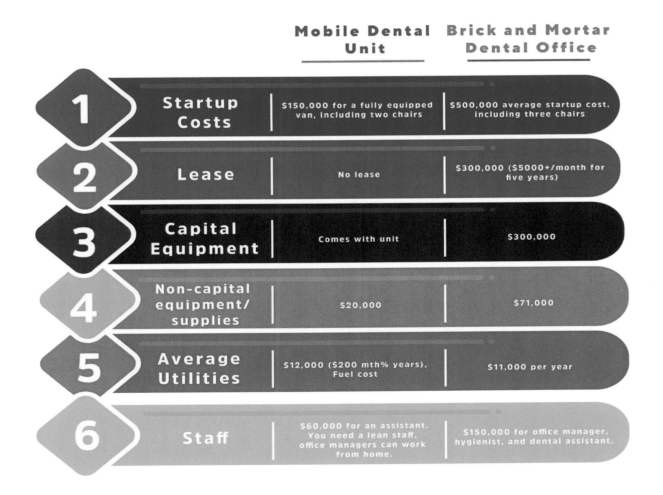

		Mobile Dental Unit	Brick and Mortar Dental Office
1	Startup Costs	$150,000 for a fully equipped van, including two chairs	$500,000 average startup cost, including three chairs
2	Lease	No lease	$300,000 ($5000+/month for five years)
3	Capital Equipment	Comes with unit	$300,000
4	Non-capital equipment/supplies	$20,000	$71,000
5	Average Utilities	$12,000 ($200 mth% years), Fuel cost	$11,000 per year
6	Staff	$60,000 for an assistant. You need a lean staff, office managers can work from home.	$150,000 for office manager, hygienist, and dental assistant.

Cost differences between mobile and office dentistry

The following are two types of dentist vans that cost between $150,000 and $300,000.

Mobile Van

A Kare Mobile Van 2.0 costs $150,000. Energy-efficient, it has a temperature-related component to keep cold things cold and hot things hot. So the temperature of your surroundings will not affect the equipment. This van is also easier to drive and operate and requires less cost to maintain. The Kare Van comes with a Kare App mobile app, which makes it convenient to schedule appointments for patients and bill insurance. The app lets you know the location of the patient. It also lets the patient know how close you are to their location and what services you offer and sends them alerts when their appointments are due.

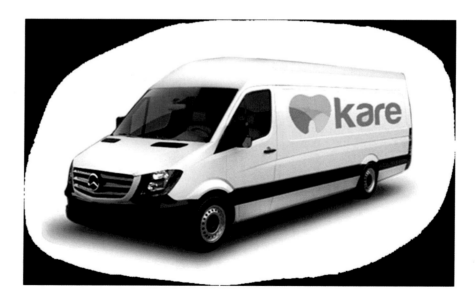

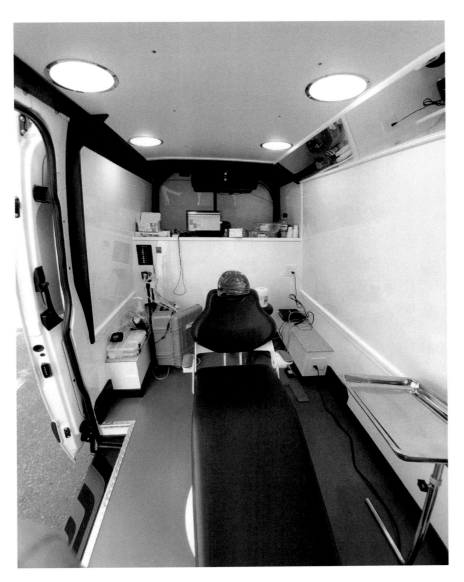

A Kare Mobile Van 2.0 is easy to drive and operate and does not cost much to maintain.

Mobile Van Clinics/Grant Program

A mobile van clinic costs $300,000. It has an efficient design and is completely set up and ready to use on arrival. It requires maintenance, insurance, a place to park, and a competent driver. However, a CDL license is not required to drive it. The van needs to be designed to allow access of the disabled. When using it, you need to develop a strategy to efficiently move and manage patients in a confined space.

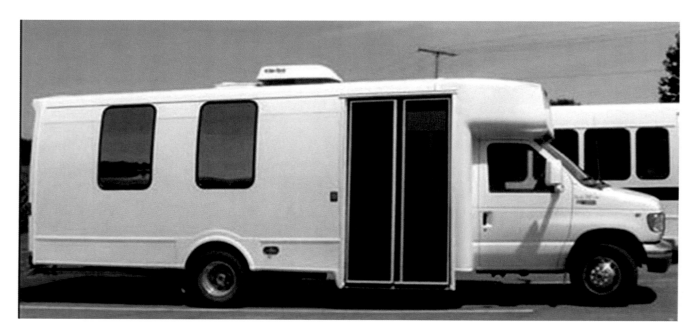

This van is completely set up and ready to use on arrival.

Challenges of Owning a Mobile Dental Unit

There are several benefits to owning a mobile dentistry practice. But you may also experience challenges, particularly in the beginning. First, as you set up the mobile clinic, you will need to purchase a van, buy equipment, and hire staff, which could be expensive. To overcome this challenge, purchase a van and equipment that costs less but is just as effective. Also some workers, such as the manager, can work from home to cut costs.

Another complication that might arise when you start your mobile dental unit is that you may need to market your services to attract patients to dentistry. This includes targeting the right demographic, putting up a website, asking patients to write testimonials, and sending patients reminders when they are due for dental appointments. Since most dentists are not trained in marketing, you can hire a professional marketer to help you promote your mobile dentistry business.

Finally you might not have a dentist traveling with you at all times. So you will need to refer challenging cases to a dentist's office.

Summary

Mobile dentistry involves dental professionals, such as dentists, dental hygienists, and dental assistants, traveling in vans with their equipment to provide care to patients near their homes. This increases the accessibility of dental care to underserved populations. Dental professionals can practice different types of mobile dentistry, including geriatric, school base, special needs, corporate, addiction recovery facilities, homebound, and whitening dentistry. One of the main advantages of operating a mobile dentistry is that operation costs are not as expensive as those of a stationary dentist's office.

However, the dental professional may experience some challenges when setting up the unit, including lack of a dentist, high start-up costs, and having to market the mobile clinic to get patients. These can be addressed by considering cost-effective alternatives, setting up a website, seeking patients' testimonials, sending your patients reminders for their appointments, and hiring a marketing professional.

11—The ABCs of Poor Oral Care in Aging Adults

Sonya Dunbar, the Geriatric Toothfairy

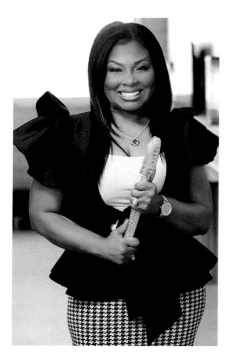

If your mouth is not healthy, your whole body is not healthy.

t is important to understand oral systemic links. The mouth is the gateway to the body. It is essential to keep the gateway clean and healthy. If your mouth is not healthy, your whole body is not healthy. Knowing the signs of unhealthy oral health is imperative as those signs can lead you to take precaution and prevention measures. Some telltale signs of unhealthy oral conditions include noticing blood in the sink after brushing or if your toothbrush is pink after brushing. These symptoms can be a sign of the early stages of gum disease. Constant bad breath and mobile teeth can also imply that you have gum disease. Gum disease can lead to or aggravate many fatal diseases. Dying from a dirty mouth is not an option! The following are the ABCs of poor oral health, a list of diseases and conditions that are associated with oral health and preventative care.

→ A: Alzheimer—Alzheimer's is directly correlated to the cause of dementia. Alzheimer's disease accounts for 60 to 80 percent of dementia cases.[51] Alzheimer's leads to poor oral care.

→ B: Blood Pressure—Poor oral health interferes with blood pressure control, specifically gum infections. Gum infections and tooth damage worsens blood pressure and interferes with hypertension treatment.[52]

→ C: Cancer—Cancer mortality rates are higher for older adults, with approximately 70 percent of all cancer deaths occurring in older adults over the age of sixty-five. Poor habits, such as smoking tobacco products, can lead to oral and throat cancers. Aged adults who do not smoke but suffer from gum disease are at risk for kidney, pancreatic, and blood cancers.[53]

→ D: Diabetes—Aged adults with diabetes have a higher chance of having periodontal (gum) disease, an infection of the gum and bone that hold the teeth in place. Periodontal disease can lead to pain, bad breath that doesn't go away, chewing difficulties, and even tooth loss.[54]

→ E: Eating Disorders—Eating disorders affect our elders' oral health. Without proper nutrition, gums and other soft tissue inside the mouth bleed easily. The glands that produce saliva swell, causing aging adults to experience chronic dry mouth. Excessive vomiting affects the teeth because strong stomach acid breaks down the tooth's enamel, which affects the color, shape, and length of teeth. The edges of the teeth become thin and break off easily.[55]

→ F: Fungus—Aging adults with weakened immunity and poor oral hygiene are more likely to get a fungal infection in the mouth. Oral fungus must be treated immediately because it can lead to health complications if it is left untreated.[56]

→ G: Gum Disease—About 68 percent of aging adults starting at the age of sixty-five or older have gum disease, leading to tooth loss. Nearly one in five adults aged sixty-five or older have lost all of their teeth due to gum disease. Complete tooth loss is twice as prevalent among adults aged seventy-five and older.[57]

→ H: Heart Disease—Heart disease and periodontitis are directly correlated. Having periodontitis increases an aging adult's risk of developing heart disease. Poor dental health increases the risk of a bacterial infection in the bloodstream, affecting the heart valves.[58]

→ I: Infection Control—According to the AAFP, infectious diseases account for a third of all deaths in people over the age of sixty-five. More than 90 percent of all deaths from pneumonia occur in people over sixty-five. Even a common infection such as influenza is far more deadly to the elderly than to others.[59]

→ J: Jaw pain—Jaw pain, also referred to as temporomandibular joint disorder (TMJ), is a condition that occurs when the joints on the side of the jaw aren't working properly. For the following reasons, older adults are generally the recipients of TMJ pain treatment.

→ K: Kidney Disease—Kidney disease is a severe health problem that affects the kidneys, heart, bones, and blood pressure. Kidney disease can be fatal if it leads to kidney failure or cardiovascular disease. Infections in the body, such as periodontal disease, can lead to kidney disease. Many people who suffer from feeble oral health also suffer from kidney disease.[60]

→ L: Leukoplakia—Leukoplakia causes white patches, or plaques, to develop on the tongue and mucosa in the mouth. Mouth irritants and irritating activities, such as smoking, often cause leukoplakia.[61]

➔ M: Malodor mouth sores—Malodor mouth sores, or tender spots in the mouth, may indicate health problems in the mouth and the rest of the body, especially if they keep returning.[62]

➔ O: Osteoporosis—Osteoporosis is a condition in which the bones become less dense and more likely to fracture. Research suggests a link between osteoporosis and bone loss in the jaw. The bone in the jaw supports and anchors the teeth. When the jawbone becomes less dense, tooth loss can occur, a common occurrence in older adults.[63]

➔ P: Pneumonia—Poor oral health in aged persons is a risk of aspiration pneumonia. The risk of aspiration pneumonia is most significant when periodontal disease, dental caries, and poor oral hygiene are compounded by swallowing disease, feeding problems, and low functional status.[64]

➔ R: Respiratory infections/Rheumatoid arthritis—The respiratory system can suffer as a result of poor oral health. Bacteria in the mouth from infected teeth and swollen gums can be breathed into the lungs or travel there through the bloodstream. Once there, the bacteria can lead to respiratory infections, pneumonia, and acute bronchitis.[65]

➔ S: Stomatitis/Thrush—Stomatitis is caused by a yeast or fungus called candida. It is not an infection that we get or pass on to others because we all have some candida in our mouths. Stomatitis, also referred to as thrush, can appear in other parts of the body, but it may be called denture stomatitis when it affects the mouth.

➔ T: Teeth Decay—Tooth decay is the softening of the tooth enamel and refers to the damage of the tooth structure caused by acids created when plaque bacteria break down sugar in the mouth. If this loss of mineral from the enamel is left untreated, a cavity, or hole in the tooth, can eventually occur.[66]

➔ U: Ulcerative gingivitis—Ulcerative gingivitis is a progressive painful infection with ulceration, swelling, and sloughing off dead tissue from the mouth and throat due to the spread of infection from the gums.[67]

→ X: Xerostomia—Xerostomia is reduced salivary flow, which can cause difficulties in tasting, chewing, swallowing, and speaking. It can also increase the chance of developing dental decay, demineralization of teeth, tooth sensitivity, and oral infections.

→ Y: Yeast/Oral thrush—Oral yeast infection is a common disease in wearers of dentures, particularly if they don't fit properly and have poor oral hygiene or a perpetually dry mouth.[68]

Summary

The mouth is the gateway to the body. Knowing the signs of an unhealthy mouth is important as these can lead you to take prevention measures. For example, symptoms of early stages of gum disease might include bleeding gums. If you notice bleeding after brushing your teeth, see a dental professional as untreated gum disease can cause other diseases, such as Alzheimer's, high blood pressure, cancer, diabetes, an eating disorder, and fungus. Other diseases that have been linked to gum disease are heart disease, infection control, jaw pain, kidney disease, leukoplakia, malodor mouth sores, osteoporosis, pneumonia, respiratory infections, stomatitis, tooth decay, ulcerative gingivitis, xeromastia, and yeast. Saving your mouth can save your life.

Epilogue

Sonya Dunbar

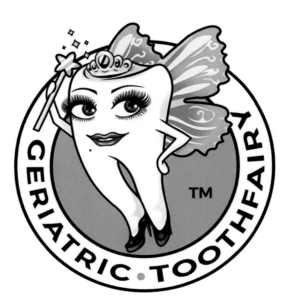

As the Geriatric Toothfairy, I have taken wings of my own. My life is dedicated to helping care for underserved communities. Luckily dentistry has grown outside of the brick-and-mortar building, and many dental professionals are now going mobile. I assist dental professionals all over the country become mobile in whatever area they choose, from pop-up dental, nursing homes, school base, drug addiction, or mobile whitening. If you want help getting into mobile dentistry, contact Sonyadunbar.org.

In 2019, Melissa Turner and I held our inaugural National Mobile and Teledentistry Conference in Orlando, Florida. We had over four hundred dental professionals, networking and growing our mobile dental community. The 2021 National Mobile and Teledentistry Conference will be held in Orlando. The 2022 conference will be in Las Vegas. For more information, visit nmdconference.com.

We also welcome you to join the American Mobile and Teledentistry Alliance. Melissa and I developed the alliance to bring more cohesiveness to mobile and teledentistry. We realize that together we are stronger. Come grow with us as we make changes in mobile and teledentistry. For more information, visit amda.net.

Until next time, stay safe and courageous!

Dr. Alisa Kauffman

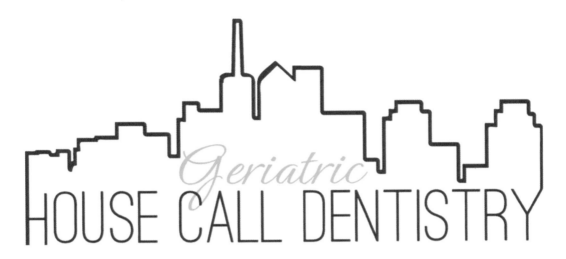

Geriatric house call dentistry is a growing field. So much has changed since I graduated from dental school in the 1980s. Most dental schools and universities today are focusing on teaching their students how to treat the differently abled and aged, and some are even teaching how to safely treat patients in their homes.

I am excited to see that Medicare has finally acknowledged that dental care is essential to overall systemic health. Oral health matters and individuals are keeping their teeth well into their nineties and hundreds. Dental implants are replacing bridges that unnecessarily cut down healthy teeth to replace one tooth that was lost, and technology is changing everything, including how we practice dentistry.

My final bit of advice is to floss the teeth you want to keep, brush, and use an oral rinse. And if you have any questions or need more product recommendations, please do not hesitate to reach out to me.

Thank you to Chris David from Syndicate Marketing for your friendship and technology support that you have given to me over the last eight years. Without your quick wit and patience, I do not think that my network could have grown so quickly. You are a genius! And thank you to Laura Hausler and Dr. Joel Berg for all your wonderful ideas that stimulate my brain.

Footnotes

1. "Glossary-common dental & periodontal terms," Periodontal Glossary, https://www.gumsurgery.com/about/periodontal-glossary/.

2. "By 2030 all baby boomers will be age 65 or older," United States Census Bureau, https://www.census.gov/library/stories/2019/12/by-2030-all-baby-boomers-will-be-age-65-or-older.html.

3. "Older adults oral health," Centers for Disease Control and Prevention, https://www.cdc.gov/oralhealth/basics/adult-oral-health/adult_older.htm.

4. Ibid.

5. J. Misachi, "What is a baby boomer?" https://www.worldatlas.com/articles/what-is-a-baby-boomer.html.

6. J. Chappelow, "Baby Boomer," https://www.investopedia.com/terms/b/baby_boomer.asp.

7. "US nursing assistants employed in nursing homes: key facts," PHI, https://phinational.org/wp-content/uploads/legacy/phi-nursing-assistants-key-facts.pdf.

8. "What you'll study in a CNA program," All Nursing Schools, https://www.allnursingschools.com/certified-nursing-assistant/degrees/#:~:text=Generally%2C%20most%20certified%20nursing%20assistant,classroom%20instruction%20and%20clinical%20training.

9. "Essential Care-Giver Guidance for Long-term Care Facilities," Minnesota Department of Health, https://www.health.state.mn.us/diseases/coronavirus/hcp/ltccaregiver.html.

10. "Depression in the Elderly," WebMD, https://www.webmd.com/depression/guide/depression-elderly#1.

11. Ibid.

12. "Oral health and mental illness: Yes, they are related," MHM Content, https://mental-health-matters.com/oral-health-and-mental-illness-yes-they-are-related/.

13. E. Meyer, "Why it's important that seniors have a social life," https://www.walkermethodist.org/blog/why-its-important-for-seniors-to-have-a-social-life.

14. L. Slack-Smith, A. Durey, and C. Scrine, "Successful ageing and oral health: incorporating dental professionals into aged care facilities," https://openresearch-repository.anu.edu.au/bitstream/1885/139320/3/Aged%20care%20Full%20report%20FINAL.pdf.

15. T. Yoneyama, M. Yoshida, T. Ohrui, et al. "Oral care reduces pneumonia in older patients in nursing homes," *J Am Geriatr Soc* 2002 50: 430–433, https://www.researchgate.net/profile/Mitsuyoshi_Yoshida/publication/11423562_Oral_care_reduces_pneumonia_in_older_patients_in_nursing_homes/links/59ed2cee4585151983ccda68/Oral-care-reduces-pneumonia-in-older-patients-in-nursing-homes.pdf.

16. E. M. Ghezzi, K. Keita, P. Deok-Young, and S. Patcharawan, "Oral healthcare systems for an ageing population: concepts and challenges," *International Dental Journal* 67: 26–33, https://onlinelibrary.wiley.com/doi/full/10.1111/idj.12343.

17. A. M. Delgado, T. Prihoda, C. Nguyen, B. Hicks, L. Smiley, and M. Taverna, "Professional caregivers' oral care practices and beliefs for elderly clients aging in place," *American Dental Hygienists' Association* 90(4)(2016): 244–248, https://jdh.adha.org/content/jdenthyg/90/4/244.full.pdf.

18. S. Peter, *Essentials of Preventive and Community Dentistry* (New Delhi: Arya (Medi) Publishing House, 2004).

19. Ibid.

20. P.A. Razak, K. J. Richard, R. P. Thankachan, K. A. Hafiz, K. N. Kumar, and K. M. Sameer, "Geriatric oral health: a review article," *Journal of international oral health* 6(6)(2014): 110, https://www.ncbi.nlm.nih.gov/pmc/articles/PMC4295446/.

21. L. Slack-Smith, A. Durey, and C. Scrine, "Successful ageing and oral health: incorporating dental professionals into aged care facilities," https://openresearch-repository.anu.edu.au/bitstream/1885/139320/3/Aged%20care%20Full%20report%20FINAL.pdf.

22. E. M. Ghezzi, K. Kobayashi, D. Y. Park, and P. Srisilapanan, "Oral healthcare systems for an ageing population: concepts and challenges," *International dental journal* 67 (2017): 26–33, https://onlinelibrary.wiley.com/doi/full/10.1111/idj.12343.

23. W.C. Gonsalves, A. S. Wrightson, and R. G. Henry, "Common oral conditions in older persons," https://www.aafp.org/afp/2008/1001/p845.html#afp20081001p845-t3.

24. "Illicit drug use," National Center for Health and Statistics, https://www.cdc.gov/nchs/fastats/drug-use-illicit.htm?CDC_AA_refVal=https%3A%2F%2Fwww.cdc.gov%2Fnchs%2Ffastats%2Fdrug-use-illegal.htm.

25. "How drug abuse affects dental health," American Addiction Centers, https://americanaddictioncenters.org/health-complications-addiction/dental-health.

26. G. K. Saini, N. D. Gupta, and K. C. Prabhat, "Drug addiction and periodontal diseases," *Journal of Indian Society of Periodontology* 17(5)(2013): 587, https://www.ncbi.nlm.nih.gov/pmc/articles/PMC3808011/.

27. H. Shekarchizadeh, M. R. Khami, S. Z. Mohebbi, H. Ekhtiari, and J. I. Virtanen, "Oral health of drug abusers: a review of health effects and care," *Iranian journal of public health* 42(9)(2013): 929, https://www.ncbi.nlm.nih.gov/pmc/articles/PMC4453891/.

28. "How drug abuse affects dental health," American Addiction Centers, https://americanaddictioncenters.org/health-complications-addiction/dental-health.

29. J. Vespa, D. M. Armstrong, L. Medina, and US Census Bureau, "Demographic turning points for the United States: Population projections for 2020 to 2060,"_https://www.census.gov/content/dam/Census/library/publications/2020/demo/p25-1144.pdf.

30. F. Müller, "Oral hygiene reduces the mortality from aspiration pneumonia in frail elders," *Journal of dental research* 94(3_suppl)(2013): 14S–16S, https://www.ncbi.nlm.nih.gov/pmc/articles/PMC4541086/.

31. Ibid.

32. L Goyal, A. Bey, N. D. Gupta, and V. K. Sharma, "Comparative evaluation of serum c-reactive protein levels in chronic and aggressive periodontitis patients and association with periodontal disease severity," *Contemp Clin Dent* 5(4)(2014): 484–488, https://www.ncbi.nlm.nih.gov/pmc/articles/PMC4229757/.

33. AA El-Solh, "Association between pneumonia and oral care in nursing home residents," *Lung* 189(2013):173–180, https://link.springer.com/article/10.1007/s00408-011-9297-0.

34. A. Holmlund, E. Lampa, and L. Lind, "Oral health and cardiovascular disease risk in a cohort of periodontitis patients," *Atherosclerosis* 262 (2017): 101–106, https://www.sciencedirect.com/science/article/abs/pii/S0021915017302125.

35. P. M. Bracci, "Oral health and the oral microbiome in pancreatic cancer: an overview of epidemiological studies," *The Cancer Journal* 23(6)(2017): 310–314, https://journals.lww.com/journalppo/fulltext/2017/11000/Oral_Health_and_the_Oral_Microbiome_in_Pancreatic.2.aspx.

36. S. A. Moghadam, M. Shirazaiy, and S. Risbaf, "The associations between periodontitis and respiratory disease," *Journal of Nepal Health Research Council* 15(1)(2017): 1–6, https://www.nepjol.info/index.php/JNHRC/article/view/18023.

37. C.-K. Chen, Y.-T. Wu, and Y.-C Chang, "Association between chronic periodontitis and the risk of Alzheimer's disease: a retrospective, population-based, matched-cohort study," *Alzheimers Res. Ther.* 9(2017): 56, doi: 10.1186/s13195-017-0282-6. https://link.springer.com/article/10.1186/s13195-017-0282-6.

38. D. Ni Chroinin, A. Montalto, S. Jahromi, N. Ingham, A. Beveridge, and P. Foltyn, "Oral health status is associated with common medical comorbidities in older hospital inpatients," *Journal of the American Geriatrics Society* 64(8)(2016): 1696–1700, https://onlinelibrary.wiley.com/doi/abs/10.1111/jgs.14247.

39. B. Kamdem, L. Seematter-Bagnoud, F. Botrugno, and B. Santos-Eggimann, "Relationship between oral health and Fried's frailty criteria in community-dwelling older persons," *BMC geriatrics* 17(1)(2017): 174, https://link.springer.com/article/10.1186/s12877-017-0568-3.

40. "Who are children with special health care needs," Child and Adolescent Health Measurement Initiative (CAHMI), http://childhealthdata.org/.

41. "Children and youth with special healthcare needs in emergencies," Centers for Disease Control and Prevention, https://www.cdc.gov/childrenindisasters/children-with-special-healthcare-needs.html.

42. "Developmental disabilities and oral health," National Institutes of Health (NIH), https://www.nidcr.nih.gov/health-info/developmental-disabilities/more-info.

43. Angelia M. Paschal, Jereme D. Wilroy, and Suzanne R. Hawley, "Unmet needs for dental care in children with special health care needs," *Preventive medicine reports* 3 (2016): 62–67, https://reader.elsevier.com/reader/sd/pii/S2211335515001709?token=7A07138AD276028144CAEC88624E68558A16FC76CEE1260030EDBC74723FEAAFE4E2AD33EC8D7342BDC91474354B71B1.

44. S. Gupta, M. Hakim, D. Patel, L. C. Stow, K. Shin, P. Timothé, and R. P. Nalliah, "Reaching Vulnerable Populations through Portable and Mobile Dentistry—Current and Future Opportunities," *Dentistry journal* 7(3)(2019): 75, https://www.mdpi.com/2304-6767/7/3/75.

45. K. Nasseh and M. Vujicic, "Dental care utilization steady among-working age adults and children, up slightly among elderly," American Dental Association, https://www.ada.org/~/media/ADA/Science%20and%20Research/HPI/Files/HPIBrief_1016_1.pdf.

46. WQ Qiu, M Dean, T Liu, et al, "Physical and mental health of homebound older adults: an overlooked population," *J Am Geriatr Soc* 58(12)(2010): 2423–2428, https://www.ncbi.nlm.nih.gov/pmc/articles/PMC3044592/.

47. P. Crete, L. D. Boyd, J. K. Fitzgerald, and L. M. LaSpina, "Access to preventive oral health services for homebound populations: A pilot program," *American Dental Hygienists' Association* 92(6)(2018): 24–32, https://scholar.google.com/scholar?hl=en&as_sdt=0%2C5&q=+Crete%2C+P.%2C+Boyd%2C+L.+D.%2C+Fitzgerald%2C+J.+K.%2C+%26+LaSpina%2C+L.+M.+%282018%29.+Access+to+preventive+oral+health+services+for+homebound+populations%3A+A+pilot+program.+American+Dental+Hygienists%27+Association%2C+92%286%29%2C+24-32.&btnG=.

48. Ibid.

49. "Whitening Survey," American Academy of Cosmetic Dentistry, https://aacd.com/proxy/files/Publications%20and%20Resources/Whitening%20Survey_Aug12(1).pdf.

50. C. M. Carey, "Tooth whitening: what we now know," *Journal of Evidence Based Dental Practice* 14(2014): 70–76, https://www.ncbi.nlm.nih.gov/pmc/articles/PMC4058574/.

51. "Tooth whitening systems," American Dental Hygienists' Association, https://www.adha.org/sites/default/files/7227_Tooth_Whitening_1.pdf.

52. "What is Alzheimer's Disease?" Alzheimer's Association, https://www.alz.org/alzheimers-dementia/what-is-alzheimers.

53. "Poor oral health linked to higher blood pressure, worse blood pressure control," American Heart Association, https://newsroom.heart.org/news/poor-oral-health-linked-to-higher-blood-pressure-worse-blood-pressure-control#:~:text=Study%20Highlights%3A,and%20interferes%20with%20hypertension%20treatment.

54. "10 health issues caused by bad oral health," Absolute Dental, https://www.absolutedental.com/blog/10-health-issues-caused-by-bad-oral-health/.

55. "Diabetes & oral health," National Institute of Dental and Craniofacial Research, https://www.nidcr.nih.gov/health-info/diabetes#:~:text=Did%20you%20know%20diabetes%20can,difficulties%2C%20and%20even%20tooth%20loss.

56. "Eating disorders," Mouth Healthy, https://www.mouthhealthy.org/en/az-topics/e/eating-disorders.

57. "4 signs of poor oral hygiene," Preferred Dental Center, https://www.preferreddentalcenter.com/4-signs-of-poor-oral-hygiene/#!.

58. "Oral health for older Americans," Centers for Disease Control and Prevention, https://www.cdc.gov/oralhealth/basics/adult-oral-health/adult_older.htm#:~:text=Oral%20health%20problems%20in%20older,5%20have%20untreated%20tooth%20decay.&text=Gum%20disease.

59. T. J. Salinas, "Will taking care of my teeth help prevent heart disease?," https://www.mayoclinic.org/healthy-lifestyle/adult-health/expert-answers/heart-disease-prevention/faq-20057986#:~:text=Gum%20disease%20(periodontitis)%20is%20associated,you%20have%20artificial%20heart%20valves.

60. "Preventing infections in the elderly," Parent Giving, https://www.parentgiving.com/elder-care/preventing-infections-elderly/.

61. "10 health issues caused by bad oral health," Absolute Dental, https://www.absolutedental.com/blog/10-health-issues-caused-by-bad-oral-health/.

62. "What to know about leukoplakia," Medical News Today, https://www.medicalnewstoday.com/articles/317689.

63. "4 signs of poor oral hygiene," Preferred Dental Center, https://www.preferreddentalcenter.com/4-signs-of-poor-oral-hygiene/#!.

64. "Oral health and bone disease," National Institutes of Health (NIH), https://www.bones.nih.gov/health-info/bone/bone-health/oral-health/oral-health-and-bone-disease.

65. M. Terpenning, "Geriatric oral health and pneumonia risk," *Clinical infectious diseases* 40(12)(2005): 1807–1810, https://academic.oup.com/cid/article/40/12/1807/314357.

66. "10 health issues caused by bad oral health," Absolute Dental, https://www.absolutedental.com/blog/10-health-issues-caused-by-bad-oral-health/.

67. "Cavities and tooth decay: symptoms, causes and treatments," Crest, https://crest.com/en-us/oral-health/conditions/cavities-tooth-decay/cavities-tooth-decay-symptoms-causes-treatment.

68. W. C. Shiel, "Medical definition of ulcerative gingivitis," https://www.medicinenet.com/ulcerative_gingivitis/definition.htm.

69. I. Gacon, J. E. Loster, and A. Wieczorek, "Relationship between oral hygiene and fungal growth in patients: users of an acrylic denture without signs of inflammatory process," *Clinical Interventions in Aging* 14(2019): 1297, https://www.ncbi.nlm.nih.gov/pmc/articles/PMC6643491/.

70. "Education You Need to Become a Certified Nursing Assistant (CNA)," https://www.allnursingschools.com/certified-nursing-assistant/degrees/.

About the Authors

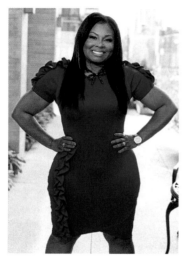

Sonya Dunbar, also known as the Geriatric Toothfairy, is a Registered Dental Hygienist, TEDx, and national public speaker guided by over 29 years of dental experience in private practice, skilled nursing facilities, and academia. Sonya and her husband, Gerald Dunbar (Navy Veterans), are the proud parents of four successful adult children. Sonya and Gerald are the owners of a thriving mobile dental company, providing comprehensive dental care to long-term care facilities. In addition, Sonya is a geriatric oral health educator and trainer. She provides informative hands-on training to Certified Nursing Assistants (CNAs) who work with aging adults. Sonya has also developed an online training course for caregivers and CNAs and works diligently to educate as many people as possible on the importance of oral health as we age. Sonya is pursuing a Ph.D. in Gerontology.

Sonya is a serial entrepreneur and successful cultural diversity workplace coach who increases cultural awareness, knowledge, and communication through interactive educational workshops. She is a known philanthropist. She is the Co-Founder of the National Mobile & Teledentistry Dental Conference, Co-Founder of The American Mobile Dentistry & Teledentistry Alliance. Sonya published author of Golden Nuggets For Life (available in English and Spanish), Co-Author of An Introduction to Mobile & Teledentistry: How Technology, Consumer Demand & Prevention Are Shaping the Future Dentistry. Sonya is the Producer of "Suave & Sassy Senior Show with Sonya," highlighting countrywide stories of aging adults doing great things and living their best life. She is also the recipient of the 2020 Philips Heart to Hands Award. As if that is not enough, the National Day Archives LLC has proclaimed November 9th of each calendar year is officially designated as "The Geriatric Toothfairy Day" and the Mayor of Jacksonville, Florida also proclaimed November 9th of each calendar year is officially dedicated as "Senior Oral Care Day."

Additional Ways to Contact Sonya Dunbar

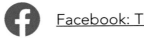 Facebook: The Geriatric Toothfairy

 Youtube: Suave & Sassy Seniors

 Instagram: Geriatric_Toothfairy

 Twitter: G Toothfairy

 Linkedin Sonya Dunbar

S.O.S Facebook Group

Dentistry Gone Wild Podcast

Website SonyaDunbar.org

Golden Nuggets for Life

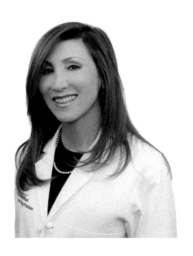

Dr. Alisa G. Kauffman received her bachelor's degree from Lehigh University in 1981 and a DMD from the University of Pennsylvania School of Dental Medicine in 1985. She maintained her private practice in New York City until 1995, when she limited her practice to geriatric house call dentistry.

In 2010, she traveled weekly between New York City and Philadelphia to the University of Pennsylvania School of Nursing, where she created a geriatric dental curriculum within a unique day program designed to keep the elderly population of West Philadelphia in their own residences while receiving a full range of daily services, including medical, dental, social services, and meals. In 2011, she was promoted to chief dental officer at the University of Pennsylvania Dental Faculty Practices, where she maintained that position until 2018, leaving to do house calls for the elderly back in New York City full time.

In addition to her house call practice, she is the director of dentistry at two skilled nursing facilities and an inventor of two oral care products that are patent pending. Dr. Kauffman is also the author of *How to Become a House Call Dentist*, a detailed step-by-step how-to guide for dentists who would like to join her growing network. Kauffman is passionate about making house calls to those who cannot get out of their homes. She believes, "When you love what you are doing, it doesn't feel like work!"

Additional Ways to Contact Alisa

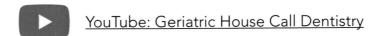 YouTube: Geriatric House Call Dentistry

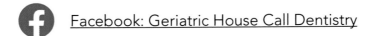 Facebook: Geriatric House Call Dentistry

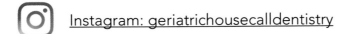 Instagram: geriatrichousecalldentistry

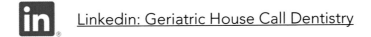 Linkedin: Geriatric House Call Dentistry

Website: www.geriatrichousecalldentistry.com

Website:www.caringandable.com

TheToothAndNothingButTheTruth.com

About the Editor

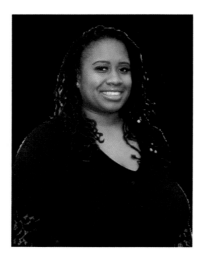

La'Risa Wilson, a published author and editor, has been writing and editing for over eight years. After working as a dental hygienist assistant, she decided to pursue and obtain a bachelor's in political science to pursue a different career. Soon after graduating, she started Letters By Reesi, a small business that provides writing and editing services for entrepreneurs and creatives. La'Risa mostly concentrates on developing impactful digital products for coaches, consultants, and influencers. She is passionate about encouraging and teaching women how to thrive financially by turning their gifts and passions into residual income.

Additional Ways to Contact La'Risa Wilson

 Facebook

Pinterest

 Linkedin

 Instagram

Website

Printed in the United States
by Baker & Taylor Publisher Services